Neurology
Emergencies

DISCLAIMER FOR CHAPTER 10

Neurology Emergencies

Jonathan A. Edlow, MD

Associate Professor of Medicine
Vice Chair, Department of Emergency Medicine
Beth Israel Deaconess Medical Center
Harvard Medical School
Boston, Massachusetts

Magdy H. Selim, MD, PhD

Associate Professor of Neurology
Co-Director, Stroke Center and Vascular Neurology
Fellowship Training Program
Beth Israel Deaconess Medical Center
Harvard Medical School
Boston, Massachusetts

OXFORD
UNIVERSITY PRESS

OXFORD
UNIVERSITY PRESS

Oxford University Press, Inc., publishes works that further
Oxford University's objective of excellence
in research, scholarship, and education.

Oxford   New York
Auckland   Cape Town   Dar es Salaam   Hong Kong   Karachi
Kuala Lumpur   Madrid   Melbourne   Mexico City   Nairobi
New Delhi   Shanghai   Taipei   Toronto

With offices in
Argentina   Austria   Brazil   Chile   Czech Republic   France   Greece
Guatemala   Hungary   Italy   Japan   Poland   Portugal   Singapore
South Korea   Switzerland   Thailand   Turkey   Ukraine   Vietnam

Published by Oxford University Press, Inc.
198 Madison Avenue, New York, New York 10016

www.oup.com

Oxford is a registered trademark of Oxford University Press.

Library of Congress Cataloging-in-Publication Data
Neurology emergencies/[edited by] Jonathan A. Edlow, Magdy H. Selim.
p. ; cm.
Includes bibliographical references and index.
ISBN 978-0-19-538858-9
1. Nervous system–Diseases. 2. Neurological intensive care. 3. Medical emergencies.
I. Edlow, Jonathan A. II. Selim, Magdy H.
[DNLM: 1. Central Nervous System Diseases–diagnosis. 2. Central Nervous System
Diseases–therapy. 3. Diagnosis, Differential. 4. Emergency Treatment–methods.
5. Neurologic Examination–methods. WL 141 N4846 2011]
RC346.N4516 2011
616.8—dc22
2010003461

616 .8 NEUROLO   2011e

Neurology emergencies

9 8 7 6 5 4 3 2

Printed in the United States of America
on acid-free paper

Contents

Series Preface

Emergency physicians care for patients with any condition that may be encountered in an emergency department. This requires that they know about a vast number of emergencies, some common and many rare. Physicians who have trained in any of the subspecialties – cardiology, neurology, OBGYN and many others – have narrowed their fields of study, allowing their patients to benefit accordingly. The Oxford University Press *Emergencies* series has combined the very best of these two knowledge bases, and the result is the unique product you are now holding. Each handbook is authored by an emergency physician and a sub-specialist, allowing the reader instant access to years of expertise in a rapid access patient-centered format. Together with evidence-based recommendations, you will have access to their tricks of the trade, and the combined expertise and approaches of a sub-specialist and an emergency physician.

Patients in the emergency department often have quite different needs and require different testing from those with a similar emergency who are in-patients. These stem from different priorities; in the emergency department the focus is on quickly diagnosing an undifferentiated condition. An emergency occurring to an in-patient may also need to be newly diagnosed, but usually the information available is more complete, and the emphasis can be on a more focused and in-depth evaluation. The authors of each *Handbook* have produced a guide for you wherever the patient is encountered, whether in an out-patient clinic, urgent care, emergency department or on the wards.

A special thanks should be extended to Andrea Seils, Senior Editor for Medicine at Oxford University Press for her vision in bringing this series to press. Andrea is aware of how new electronic media have impacted the learning process for physician-assistants, medical students, residents and fellows, and at the same time she if a firm believer in the value of the printed word. This series contains the proof that such a combination is still possible in the rapidly changing world of information technology.

Over the last twenty years, the Oxford Handbooks have become an indispensible tool for those in all stages of training throughout the world. This new series will, I am sure, quickly grow to become the standard reference for those who need to help their patients when faced with an emergency.

Jeremy Brown, MD
Series Editor
Associate Professor of Emergency Medicine
The George Washington University Medical Center

Preface

Twenty-first-century medicine has been marked by, among other things, the growth of various specialties, each with its unique perspective on any given patient. This is particularly true for patients suffering from acute neurological emergencies where emergency physicians, neurologists, radiologists, and neurosurgeons are often involved in their care. There is overlap between when the emergency physicians' work is over and the neurologists' starts. Wherever this line may be drawn, however, and it might be different in a small community hospital than in a tertiary care center, the best care and outcomes undoubtedly result from maximal cooperation and coordination between the various specialties.

Neurology Emergencies represents this teamwork in that each chapter is co-written by authors representing both the emergency medicine and neurology perspectives. To further ensure a balanced presentation that is useful to medical students and to physicians from both specialties, one editor is an emergency physician and the other is a neurologist. We have tried to create a book that will be as useful to physicians seeing patients in the emergency department as to those caring for patients on the medical or neurological wards and intensive care units.

We have purposefully focused on the acute patient. We start by covering how the neurological examination can be used to localize the problem. And because patients arrive with symptoms, not diagnoses, we then cover the various common acute presentations of these patients. Other chapters cover specific problems that are more diagnosis based, such as traumatic brain injury, stroke, and seizures. Because neuroimaging has become such an important part of the management of neurological emergencies, each chapter is illustrated with relevant computed tomography, magnetic resonance, and vascular studies, as well as other images, algorithms, and charts to clarify and supplement the text.

Each chapter is presented in a way such that it can be used during a busy shift or to review the information afterward. We hope that medical students, emergency physicians, neurologists, internists, family practitioners, critical care physicians, and hospitalists will find this book useful.

Acknowledgments

We would like to thank our wives, Pam Edlow and Kim Curtis, for putting up with the additional work and deadlines imposed by this project. We would also like to thank the staff at Oxford University Press, especially Andrea Seils and Staci Hou, for their assistance in bringing this project along. Additionally, we would like to thank Dr. Jeremy Brown for his role in initiating this series of books and this particular installment. Last, we would like to thank our house staff and our patients, who are major driving forces behind our work.

Contributors

Frank W. Drislane, MD
Professor of Neurology
Harvard Medical School
Neurologist, Comprehensive
Epilepsy Center
Beth Israel Deaconess
Medical Center
Boston, MA

Jonathan A. Edlow, MD
Associate Professor of Medicine
Vice Chair,
Department of Emergency
Medicine
Beth Israel Deaconess
Medical Center
Harvard Medical School
Boston, MA

Michael Ganetsky, MD
Clinical Instructor in Medicine
Department of Emergency
Medicine
Harvard Medical School
Beth Israel Deaconess
Medical Center
Boston, MA

Romergryko G. Geocadin, MD
Director, Neurosciences
Critical Care Division
Johns Hopkins Medical
Institutions
Associate Professor, Neurology,
Anesthesiology
Critical Care Medicine &
Neurosurgery
Johns Hopkins University
School of Medicine
Baltimore, MD

Carl A. Germann, MD, FACEP
Assistant Professor
Tufts University School of
Medicine
Boston, MA
and
Department of Emergency
Medicine
Maine Medical Center
Portland, ME

Joshua N. Goldstein, MD, PhD, FAAEM, FAHA
Assistant Professor
Department of Emergency Medicine
Harvard Medical School
Massachusetts General Hospital
Boston, MA

J. Stephen Huff, MD
Associate Professor of Emergency Medicine and Neurology
Department of Emergency Medicine
University of Virginia
Charlottesville, VA

David S. Liebeskind, MD
Associate Professor of Neurology
Neurology Director, Stroke Imaging
Co-Medical and Co-Technical Director, UCLA Cerebral Blood Flow Laboratory
Program Director, Stroke and Vascular Neurology Residency
Associate Neurology Director, UCLA Stroke Center
Los Angeles, CA

Scott A. Marshall, MD
Major, US Army Medical Corps
Clinical Fellow, Neurosciences Critical Care
Johns Hopkins University School of Medicine
Baltimore, MD
and
Assistant Professor
Department of Neurology
Uniformed Services University of the Health Sciences
Bethesda, MD

Daniel C. McGillicuddy, MD
Associate Director of ED Clinical Operations
BIDMC Department of Emergency Medicine
Assistant Residency Director
BIDMC Harvard Affiliated Emergency Medicine Residency
Harvard Medical School
Boston, MA

John E. McGillicuddy, MD
Emeritus Professor of Neurosurgery
Department of Neurosurgery
University of Michigan School of Medicine
Ann Arbor, MI
and
Clinical Professor of Neurosurgery
Division of Neurosurgery
Department of Neurological Sciences
Medical University of South Carolina
Charleston, SC

Barnett R. Nathan, MD
Associate Professor of Neurology and Internal Medicine
Department of Neurology
Division of Neurocritical Care
University of Virginia
Charlottesville, VA

Hardin A. Pantle, MD
Department of Emergency Medicine
Johns Hopkins University
Baltimore, MD

Radoslav Raychev, MD
Neurovascular Fellow
UCLA Stroke Center
Los Angeles, CA

Jonathan Rosand, MD, MSc
Director of Fellowship Training
in Vascular and Critical Care
Neurology
Massachusetts General Hospital
Brigham and Women's Hospital
Associate Professor of Neurology
Harvard Medical School
Boston, MA

Magdy H. Selim, MD, PhD
Associate Professor of
Neurology
Co-Director, Stroke Center
and Vascular Neurology
Fellowship Training Program
Beth Israel Deaconess
Medical Center
Harvard Medical School
Boston, MA

Nicholas J. Silvestri, MD
Assistant Professor of
Neurology
Department of Neurology
State University of New York
at Buffalo
School of Medicine and
Biomedical Sciences
Buffalo, NY

Sidney Starkman, MD
Professor of Emergency
Medicine and Neurology
UCLA
Director, Emergency Neurology
Program
Co-Director, UCLA Stroke
Center
Los Angeles, CA

Chapter 1

Approach to the Neurological Patient

Magdy H. Selim and Jonathan A. Edlow

1

Where is the lesion? Establishing the correct diagnosis in patients with neurological complaints largely depends on the anatomic localization of the patient's symptoms and signs as well as how those findings evolve over time. Neurological complaints lend themselves to differential diagnosis based on anatomical localization of the responsible lesion. Detailed history and examination, together with presumptive anatomical localization, can help to narrow the differential diagnosis and to direct the choice of various diagnostic studies to confirm the diagnosis. This chapter provides a brief introduction to the principles of neurological examination and anatomical localization.

The history should direct components of the neurological examination that must be evaluated with special attention. The pearls of neurological examination and history for various neurological conditions are provided in subsequent chapters. However, certain principles of history and examination warrant emphasis here.

- The rate of onset and time course of neurological complaints can provide clues to the underlying etiology. For example, the differential diagnosis of sudden and acute visual loss is different from that associated with more insidious and gradual onset of visual loss. Abrupt and acute onset often points to a vascular cause, whereas subacute onset tends to indicate an infectious or inflammatory cause, and an insidious and progressive course indicates a neoplastic process.
- A good history often points to the localization. If localization is still not clear after a careful history, do not begin the examination yet. Take a better history!

Components of the Neurological Examination

The main components of the neurological examination are as follows:

- Assess mental status, with particular attention to level of consciousness and attention.
- Complete language testing requires assessment of ALL of the following elements: (1) Fluency, (2) Comprehension, (3) Naming, (4) Repetition, (5) Reading, and (6) Writing.
  - Reading and writing should always be tested in patients whose fluency, naming, repetition, and comprehension are questionable. Aphasic patients will often have difficulties with reading and writing. This is important because incomplete

testing of language functions could lead to mislabeling aphasic patients as being confused.

- Assess cranial nerves II-XII. Testing for the olfactory nerve function (CN I) is not routinely done.
- Do a motor examination, including muscle tone and power, and presence or absence of muscle atrophy or facsiculations (visible twitches).
- Check coordination, including finger-to-nose and heel-to-shin tests, and rapid alternating movements.
- Examine reflexes, including deep tendon and plantar reflexes.
- Check sensations, including primary (light touch, pinprick, temperature, vibration, and joint position) and cortical (graphesthesia, stereognosis, and double simultaneous stimulation) sensory modalities.
  - Sensory testing is often the least reliable part of the examination. The key to an informative sensory exam is to know what you are looking for and to be aware that the patient's cooperation diminishes with repeated testing. Start the sensory examination by getting right to the point.

- Assess gait and stance, including Romberg's test and tandem walking.
  - Testing for gait and stance is an important component of the neurological examination that is often overlooked during emergency evaluation. It is a good screening test to assess the overall neurological function, and it should be performed on all neurological patients in the emergency department, whenever possible.

Depending on the clinical situation, some portions of this examination will be more important than others. For example, in assessing language, it may be important to test all the components in some patients, because abnormalities of language that are not associated with typical lateralizing motor or cranial nerve findings are one important cause of misdiagnosis. In patients who appear confused, a more complete assessment of the individual components of the language exam is helpful.

Neuroanatomical Localization

Some knowledge of neuroanatomy is essential for correct localization. For simplicity, the first step in localizing neurological lesions should be to determine if it is a central or upper motor neuron lesion (i.e., in the brain or spinal cord) vs. a peripheral or low motor neuron lesion (i.e., muscle or nerve).

▶ The hallmark of upper motor neuron lesions is hyperreflexia with or without increased muscle tone.

- Central (upper motor neuron) lesions should be localized to:
  - Brain:
    - Cortical brain (frontal, temporal, parietal, or occipital lobes)
    - Subcortical brain structures (corona radiata, internal capsule, basal ganglia, or thalamus)
    - Brainstem (medulla, pons, or midbrain)
    - Cerebellum
  - Spinal cord:
    - Cervicomedullary junction
    - Cervical
    - Thoracic
    - Lumbosacral

▶ The hallmark of lower motor neuron (LMN) lesion is decreased muscle tone, leading to flaccidity and hyporeflexia.

- Peripheral (LMN) lesions should be localized to:
  - Anterior horn cells
  - Nerve root(s)
  - Plexus
  - Peripheral nerve
  - Neuromuscular junction
  - Muscle

Figures 1.1 and 1.2 show various cortical and subcortical brain regions. Table 1.1 lists the general principles for localization of lesions in the brain.

The following pearls can help to differentiate cortical from subcortical brain lesions:

- A lesion localizing to the left hemisphere that does not affect language functions is more likely to be subcortical.
- The presence of cortical sensory deficits points to a cortical, most likely parietal, lesion.
- Weakness resulting from cortical lesions often involves the face and arm, much more than the leg, that is, cortical lesions tend to cause an incomplete hemiparesis. In contrast, subcortical lesions involving the internal capsule or basal ganglia tend to cause a complete hemiparesis.
  - An exception, are lesions involving the frontal cortex within the anterior cerebral artery territory in which case weakness often

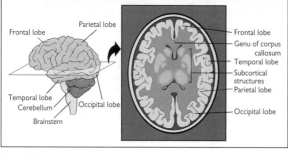

Figure 1.1 Lobes of the brain.

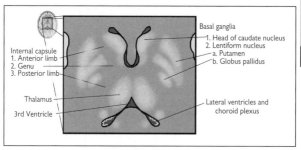

Figure 1.2 Subcortical structures of the brain.

involves the legs and deltoids and tends to spare the face and other muscle groups.

Figures 1.3, 1.4, and 1.5 show the brainstem. Table 1.2 lists the general principles for localization of lesions in these areas.

▶ The hallmark of brainstem lesions is involvement of the cranial nerves and the presence of crossed-findings, that is, cranial nerve abnormalities are contralateral to observed motor weakness in the limbs.

• The presence of cranial nerves abnormalities, other than CN VII, and long tract signs often point to a lesion in the brainstem.

• Sudden change in the level of consciousness, together with the presence of pupillary abnormalities and involuntary limb

Table 1.1 Localization of Brain Lesions

Location	Symptoms	Signs
Frontal lobe • Anterior (prefrontal) portion	• Language and behavioral changes (depression, abulia, disinhibition). • Incontinence	• Expressive-type aphasia with preserved repetition (transcortical motor aphasia), in dominant hemispheric lesions • Extinction to double simultaneous sensory stimuli and neglect,* especially in nondominant hemispheric lesions
Posterior portion	Weakness and language changes	• Contralateral weakness (leg greater than arm) • Increased tone • Grasp reflex • Buccofacial apraxia† • Transient aphasia or mutism
Temporal lobe	• Language, behavioral, and cognitive changes • Hearing loss with bilateral lesions (rare)	• Receptive aphasia • Agitated delirium (nondominant hemisphere) • Short-term memory impairment • Cortical deafness (rare)
Parietal lobe	• Language and visual changes	• Weakness (arm, especially hand, greater than face and leg) • Aphasia • Constructional, dressing, and ideomotor apraxia‡ • Anosagnosia§ • Extinction and neglect • Impairment of cortical sensory modalities • Balint's syndrome (oculomotor apraxia, simultanagnosia, and optic ataxia) with bilateral parieto-occipital lesions
Occipital lobe	• Visual, behavioral, and language changes	• Hemianopia • Cortical blindness and confabulations with bilateral lesions (Anton's syndrome) • Alexia without agraphia and color anomia (dominant hemisphere) • Visual agnosia‖ • Balint's syndrome • Agitated delerium
Corona radiata	• Weakness and sensory changes	• Patchy weakness • Impaired primary sensations

Table 1.1 (Continued)

Location	Symptoms	Signs
Internal capsule/ Basal ganglia	• Weakness	• Weakness (face, arm, and leg are equally affected) • Language is usually intact. However, some patients may develop aphasia with lesions involving the dominant basal ganglionic structures.
Thalamus	• Sensory and behavioral changes	• Impaired contralateral primary sensory modalities • Altered level of consciousness with bilateral lesions • Language is usually intact. However, some patients may develop aphasia with lesions involving the dominant basal ganglionic structures. • Hemibalismus may be seen with involvement of the subthalamic nuclei (rare).

* Failing to be aware of objects or people to their left in extrapersonal space.

†Inability to perform voluntary movements of the larynx, pharynx, mandible, tongue, lips, and cheeks, while automatic or reflexive control of these structures is preserved.

‡Apraxia refers to loss of the ability to execute or carry out learned purposeful movements, despite having the desire and the physical ability to perform the movements.

§The person is unaware of or denies the existence of his or her disability.

‖Impairment in the recognition of aspects of the visual world not due to an impairment in elementary components of vision, such as visual acuity.

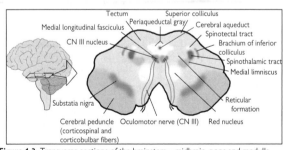

Figure 1.3 Transverse sections of the brainstem—midbrain, pons and medulla.

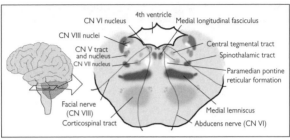

Figure 1.4 Transverse sections of the brainstem—midbrain, pons and medulla.

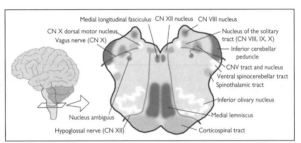

Figure 1.5 Transverse sections of the brainstem—midbrain, pons and medulla.

movements point to bilateral thalamic and brainstem involvement (top of the basilar syndrome).

Figure 1.6 shows a transverse section of the spinal cord (cervical level). Table 1.3 lists the general aspects of localization in the spinal cord.

▶ The hallmark of spinal cord lesion is hyperreflexiadistal weakness, bowel and bladder dysfunction, and the presence of a sensory level.

● Quadriparesis or paraparesis without facial weakness point to a spinal cord lesion. However, high cervical (C2–C4) and foramen magnum lesions may also result in facial numbness, ipsilateral Horner's, and ipsilateral weakness of the tongue and trapezius muscle.

● Ipsilateral facial numbness, Horner's, and tongue and trapezius weakness may be seen with upper cervical lesions near the foramen magnum.

Table 1.2 Localization of Brainstem Lesions

Location	Symptom	Sign
Midbrain	• Diplopia, weakness, and abnormal movements (tremors or ataxia)	• Impaired upward gaze • CN III or IV palsy • Contralateral hemiparesis or ataxia
Pons	• Speech and swallowing difficulties, weakness, sensory changes, and diplopia	• Dysarthria • Ipsilateral facial (CN VII) weakness – total or partial* • CN VI palsy • Horner's syndrome† • Contralateral hemiparesis or sensory loss • Impaired horizontal gaze • Nystagmus • Ataxia • Quadriplegia with bilateral lesions affecting the basis pontis
Medulla	• Dizziness, vertigo, difficulty swallowing, hiccups, nausea and vomiting, and unsteadiness	• Horner's syndrome • CN IX, X, and XII involvement • Ataxia • Ipsilateral sensory loss (face and body) • Hemiplegia may be seen with medial lesions (rare)
Cerebellum	• Unsteadiness and dizziness, nausea, and vomiting	• Ipsilateral ataxia of the limbs • Gait ataxia • Ipsilateral CN VI-like palsy (rare) • Nystagmus • Dysarthria

*Complete facial weakness and contralateral hemiplegia point to a pontine lesion.
†Horner's syndrome is always ipsilateral to the lesion.

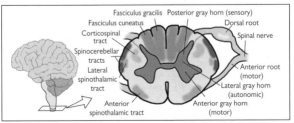

Figure 1.6 Transverse section of the spinal cord (cervical level).

Table 1.3 Localization of spinal cord lesions

Anterior cord	Weakness Sensory changes Changes in bowel and bladder functions	Upper and lower motor weakness Spinothalamic sensory loss, while sparing the posterior column sensations Sphincter dysfunction
Central cord (most commonly affects the cervical region)	Weakness Sensory changes (including burning dysesthesias)	LMN paraparesis and wasting and fasciculations of the arms Sensory loss in a "shawl" or "cape" distribution
Posterior cord	Sensory changes Segmental "band-like" sensory changes	Loss of vibration and joint position sensations
Conus medullaris	Sacral sensory changes Back or buttocks pain Changes of bowel or bladder functions	Sensory loss in the saddle area Sphincter dysfunction Weakness in L5/S1-innervated (foot and ankle) muscles
Cauda equina	Sensory changes Changes in bowel or bladder functions	Sensory loss in multiple bilateral dermatomes Sphincter dysfunction Paraparesis

Table 1.4 Localization of lower motor neuron lesions

Location	Symptoms	Signs
Anterior horn	Flaccid weakness	Muscle wasting and weakness Fasciculations No sensory loss
Nerve root and plexus	Pain Weakness and sensory changes (usually limited to a single limb)	Weakness Sensory loss (radicular or plexus distribution) Hyporeflexia
Nerve	Weakness Sensory changes	Focal weakness (can be distal in polyneuropathy) Hyporeflexia Sensory loss
Neuromuscular junction	Fluctuating weakness Intermittent diplopia or slurred speech	Positive tensilon test Weakness on repetitive testing No sensory loss
Muscle	Weakness Difficulty climbing stairs or getting out of a car Muscle aches and cramps	Proximal weakness

- Hyperreflexia due to a brain lesion may be associated with an exaggerated jaw jerk, which could help to differentiate it from hyperreflexia of spinal origin.

Table 1.4 summarizes localization in the LMN system.

- Proximal symmetrical weakness without sensory loss often points to a muscle disease (myopathy). Weakness confined to one side of the body or one limb is seldom caused by a myopathy.
- Fatigability, that is, weakness worsens with use and improves with rest, is the hallmark of lesions affecting the neuromuscular junction.
- Unlike muscle and neuromuscular junction lesions, weakness caused by peripheral nerve lesions is often distal and asymmetric, and sensory changes are almost always present.

Suggested Reading

Brazis P, Masdeu J, Biller J. (Eds.). *Localization in Clinical Neurology*. Philadelphia: Lippincott Williams & Wilkins; 2007.

Waxman S. (Ed.). *Clinical Neuroanatomy*. New York: McGraw-Hill; 2003.

Chapter 2

Presenting Symptoms

Magdy H. Selim and Jonathan A. Edlow

13

Introduction

It is obvious that when patients see clinicians, they present with symptoms, not diagnoses. Therefore, a patient presents not with a subarachnoid hemorrhage, but with an acute severe headache. They present with dysarthria and dizziness, not a cerebellar infarction. In most of this book, we have approached neurological emergencies by diagnosis or diagnostic groups. In this chapter, we focus on an algorithmic diagnostic approach to various presenting neurological symptoms.

Because this is a book on neurological emergencies, we will focus on acute presentations rather than chronic ones. Furthermore, we will focus on cannot-miss diagnoses. This refers to diagnoses or pathological conditions which are life, limb, vision, or brain threatening and for which a good treatment exists. Whether in the emergency department, the intensive care unit or the neurology in-patient ward, it is this sort of focus that must be front of mind when evaluating patients with neurological emergencies. If these cannot-miss diagnoses are missed, it is quite likely there will be a bad outcome.

Finally, many of these chief complaints are among the most common in all of medicine. The proportion of cannot-miss causes of headache, for example, or dizziness is very low. Working up all patients with these symptoms would be a waste of time and other resources. Therefore, the history and physical examination are very important in deciding which patients with these various symptoms require further emergent or urgent evaluation and which can be evaluated on a more leisurely outpatient schedule is critical.

Altered Mental Status

For simplicity, sudden alteration in mental status can be divided into:

- Delirium or encephalopathy: characterized by (often fluctuating) confusion, inattention, alteration of arousal, and global cognitive dysfunction.
- Coma refers to unconsciousness with impairment of awareness and wakefulness.

Causes and Localization

- Delirium (encephalopathy) often results from widespread dysfunction of cortical and subcortical structures due to a variety of reasons summarized in Table 2.1.

Table 2.1 **Causes of Delirium (Encephalopathy)**
Infections: Systemic or CNS. CNS infections should be considered in immunocompromised patients
Metabolic abnormalities, including electrolyte disorders, uremia, hepatic or pancreatic dysfunction
Endocrine abnormalities, such as thyroid dysfunction and adrenal insufficiency
Nutritional deficiencies, such as vitamin B1 deficiency (Wernicke's encephalopathy)
Drugs and alcohol intoxication
Medications, such as steroids, anticholinergics, tricyclics, and antihistamines
Brain focal lesions, such as intracerebral hemorrhage, ischemic stroke, or tumors involving the parietal or occipital regions can result in agitations and delirium-like state
Head trauma with or without secondary hemorrhage or contusion
Seizures and postictal state
Hypertensive encephalopathy
Hypoxic-ischemic encephalopathy

15

Table 2.2 **Causes of Coma**
Focal brain lesions involving the brainstem or cerebellum
Obstructive hydrocephalus or other causes of increased intracranial pressure
Nonconvulsive status epilepticus or postictal state
Metabolic and electrolyte disturbances
Hypothyroidism
Hypoxic-ischemic injury, such as cardiac arrest

- The most common cause is systemic infections, such as urosepsis, particularly in elderly patients.
- Coma can result from bilateral supratentorial hemispheric lesions, infratentorial lesions that impair the reticular activating system in the brainstem or thalamus, or widespread dysfunction of the brain.
  - Most causes of encephalopathy can also cause coma.
  - The most common cause of coma is related to sedatives and toxins. Table 2.2 lists the most common cause of coma.

Presentation and Evaluation

- The presentation of altered mental status is variable and ranges from drowsiness (the patient can be aroused briefly by verbal command), stupor (the patients only responds to noxious stimulation but not to voice), and delirium, to the extreme state of coma.
- The hallmark of delirium and encephalopathy is the patient's inability to maintain attention to the environment. These patients are often disoriented. They may be agitated or somnolent. Visual and auditory hallucinations may be present, and speech is often incoherent.
  - Aphasia, especially Wernicke's type, is often mistaken for confusion. Detailed language examination and clear sensorium provide clues to the correct diagnosis.
  - Strokes involving the occipital and parietal regions may present with agitations and may be mistaken for delirium.
- Although examination of the delirious and encephalopathic patients is challenging and history is often limited, one needs to pay special attention to the following:
  - History: Some historical features can provide clues to the etiology. For example:
    - Headache may indicate an intracranial cause, such as hemorrhage.
    - Eliciting history of drug and medications use, particularly, anticholinergics, can be helpful.
  - Funduscopic examination: Hypertensive changes could indicate hypertensive encephalopathy, or papilledema could be a sign of increased intracranial pressure (ICP).
  - Pupils:
    - Fixed and dilated pupils could indicate anticholinergic toxicity or brain herniation.
    - Dilated but reactive pupils could indicate intoxication with cocaine, amphetamine, or other sympathomimetics.
    - Small pinpoint pupils could indicate intoxication with opioids or pontine dysfunction.
    - Coma in the presence of reactive pupils often indicates a toxic-metabolic etiology.
  - Eye movements: Eye movements should be tested by "doll's eye maneuver", especially if no spontaneous eye movements are detected by inspection. **NB: This should only be done if there is no suspicion of any trauma that could be associated with a cervical spine lesion.**
    - Asymmetric eye movements often indicate structural, rather than toxic-metabolic causes.

- Conjugate deviation of the eyes raises the possibility of an ipsilateral cerebral hemispheric lesion, contralateral thalamic or pontine lesion, or seizures arising from a contralateral hemispheric lesion.
- Abnormal movements:
  - Myoclonic movements could indicate metabolic abnormalities, seizures, or hypoxic-ischemic injury.
  - Tremors may be seen in hyperthyroidism, intoxication with sympathomimetics or alcohol, or drug withdrawal.
  - Occasionally, myoclonic- or seizure-like movements may be seen in patients with acute basilar thrombosis! These are often mistaken for seizures and postictal encephalopathy. Abnormal eye movements or papillary abnormalities should provide clues to the diagnosis.
  - Posturing usually indicates a structural lesion. However, it may occasionally be seen with severe metabolic disorders.
- Motor response: Assess spontaneous movements of the limbs and those movements that are elicited in response to painful stimulation.
  - Asymmetric motor findings suggest structural lesions, until proven otherwise.
- General physical examination:
  - The presence of fever or hypothermia may point to an underlying infection; neck rigidity may be indicative of a meningitis or encephalitis, or subarachnoid hemorrhage (SAH).
  - Blood pressure: Hypertension may indicate an underlying hypertensive encephalopathy or it may be the cause of a stroke or an intracranial hemorrhage; hypotension may indicate shock.
  - Check for signs of head trauma.
  - Inspect skin for signs of intravenous drug use or liver disease.
- The following distinct conditions are worth mentioning:
  - Transient Global Amnesia: Patients often present with acute confusion, characterized by acute memory loss (mostly antegrade with a variable degree of retrograde amnesia) and tendency to repeat the same questions over and over. Examination is usually normal with intact consciousness and attention. The episode of amnesia is usually self-limited, lasting for several hours. This condition is usually seen in middle-aged, commonly hypertensive, patients. Its pathogenesis is poorly understood. Possible explanations include: transient ischemia, focal seizures, or a migrainous phenomenon.

- Top of the basilar syndrome: This is caused by embolism into the distal basilar artery and its branches, and subsequent infarctions in the thalami, midbrain, pons, cerebellum, and occipital lobes. Patients may appear confused and hypersomnolent. Ocular abnormalities are very common and include: limitations of vertical eye movements, visual defects, skewed deviation, pupillary abnormalities, and third and fourth cranial nerve palsies. Occasionally, involuntary movements of the limbs occur, and may be mistaken for seizures.
- Locked-in Syndrome: This occurs in patients with infarction of the base of the pons involving both corticospinal and corticobulbar tracts. Patients, therefore, are quadriplegic and unable to speak. They also lose their ability to move the eyes horizontally. As a result, they appear unresponsive. However, consciousness and cognition are intact, and they are able to respond to yes/no questions appropriately by moving their eyes up or down.

Investigations

- Laboratory studies, including complete blood cell count, serum glucose, urine analysis, blood gases, and toxicology screen, will identify most potential infectious and metabolic causes.
- Brain neuroimaging (CT scan or MRI) will identify most focal brain lesions.
  - MRI may be useful in detecting HSV encephalitis; diffuse white matter disease, such as acute demyelinating encephalomyelitis or leukoencephalopathy; small multiple bihemispheric lesions; or brainstem infarcts not seen on CT scan.
- Electrocardiogram will rule out an arrhythmia or cardiac ischemia.
- Electroencephalogram may be helpful to rule out ongoing seizures or nonconvulsive status.
- Lumbar puncture may be indicated in cases in which there is suspicion for encephalitis or subarachnoid hemorrhage (SAH).

Acute Headache and Neck Pain

Causes and Localization

Primary headache disorders—migraine and tension-type headaches—are incredibly common and represent the large majority of acute headaches. Even in an acuity-skewed emergency department population, patients with cannot-miss causes of headache (see Table 2.3) probably account for less than 5 percent of patients with headache. Sorting out which patients with an acute headache require testing beyond history and physical can be difficult.

Table 2.3 Headache – Cannot-Miss Causes
Subarachnoid hemorrhage
Meningitis and encephalitis
Acute stroke (ischemic and hemorrhagic)
Cranio-cervical artery dissection
Cerebral venous sinus thrombosis
Pituitary apoplexy
Temporal arteritis
Acute narrow-angle closure glaucoma
Idiopathic intracranial hypertension (pseudotumor cerebri)
Spontaneous intracranial hypotension
Carbon monoxide poisoning
Hypertensive emergencies
Mass lesions • Abscess (brain and parameningeal) • Tumor • Hematoma (subdural, epidural and intraparenchymal) • Colloid cyst of the third ventricle

There are some situations in which the decision is easy. For example, headache patients with new focal neurological deficits or an abnormal mental status obviously need further testing to determine the reason. By logical extension, this applies to headache patients with other new physical examination findings that suggest a serious cause. Examples of this include a red eye with corneal edema suggesting acute narrow-angle closure glaucoma, or a tender nodular superficial temporal artery suggesting temporal arteritis.

In other situations, the history or physical examination may be so classic and compelling that the need for further work-up is also clear. A patient with fever, headache, and true meningismus suggests meningitis. An elderly patient on warfarin with minor head trauma and increasing headache suggests a subdural hematoma. A hypertensive patient with a worst-of-life headache that began abruptly during sexual intercourse and is associated with syncope, vomiting, and neck pain suggests an SAH.

However, there is another group of headache patients whose physical examinations are normal and whose presentation is not a classic one. In these patients the physician must carefully search for clues in the history, physical examination, and epidemiological context to decide whom to evaluate with other tests, such as brain imaging, lumbar puncture, and others. It is important to note that location of the headache is of relatively little localizing value, although the presence of occipital headache is somewhat more worrisome than others. Pure neck pain, when acute and atraumatic, also suggests a carotid or vertebral dissection or an SAH. However, any cause of headache can be perceived as neck pain. Cervical epidural abscess, tumor, or hematoma can also present with neck pain. This chapter will not discuss cervical spine trauma.

Presentation and Evaluations

- The cornerstone of diagnosis is the history and physical examination—especially the head, eye, ear, nose, and throat (HEENT) and neurological portions of the exam.
- The most important aspects of the history for headache patients are the severity, the rapidity of onset, the quality of the pain, and the presence of various associated symptoms.
- A careful neurological exam is important. Rapid onset, or thunderclap headache has a long differential diagnosis, but approximately 15 percent of thunderclap headache patients who have a normal neurological examination will have a serious cause of headache. This percentage is much higher if the neurological exam is abnormal.
- The fundoscopic exam should be done in all patients with headache.
- With respect to quality, in most patients with serious secondary causes of headache, the quality of the pain is different from that of prior headaches.
- Remember that to give a definitive diagnosis of migraine or tension headache, multiple episodes are required (5 for migraine and 10 for tension). Therefore, these primary headache disorders can never be conclusively diagnosed after a "first, worst" headache.
- Associated symptoms such as syncope, diplopia, seizure, and any other neurological symptom suggest a secondary cause. Vomiting, while common with migraine, should also arouse suspicion, especially if the patient has never vomited with prior headaches.
- As a general rule, the location of the headache is not very useful in distinguishing the cause. That said, and all other things being equal, posterior or occipital neck pain is more suggestive of a serious problem.

Investigations

- Most patients with headache do not need anything more than a history and physical examination.
- Always try to distinguish the current headache from prior ones. When was the last time that the patient had to go to an ED for

a headache? Does the patient usually vomit with their migraines? In what ways does this headache feel different from prior ones? What objective testing has the patient had? If there is a diagnosis of migraine, tension,, or sinus headaches, how was that diagnosis established?

- Patients who have an abnormal physical exam need some other test(s) to determine the etiology of headache and of the exam findings.
- Noncontrast CT scanning is an excellent test for acute hemorrhage in the parenchyma, subdural, and epidural spaces; for SAH, its sensitivity is time dependent (very good early but decays over the course of time from the hemorrhage).
- Although some processes (e.g., brain abscess and some tumors) may not show up on a noncontrast CT scan, most that are large enough to cause headache will show some secondary findings (e.g., midline shift, vasogenic edema, or some mass effect).
- In patients being evaluated for SAH with negative CT scans, a lumbar puncture (LP) should be done looking for blood and/or xanthochromia.
- In occasional patients, MRI, with arterial or venous imaging may be needed. These diagnostic considerations include cervico-cranial arterial dissections, cerebral venous sinus thrombosis, pituitary apoplexy, and spontaneous intracranial hypotension.

Clinical Pearls

- It is always important to know the limitations of the tests that one is performing. CT may be falsely negative with an acute SAH. If the wrong sequences are acquired for a MRI (diffusion-weighted images are not obtained), a stroke might be missed. Xanthochromia may be absent in an SAH during the first 12 hours.
- The presence of venous pulsations on fundoscopic exam strongly predicts normal ICP.
- A favorable response to any analgesic used for a headache does not predict a benign etiology; this includes a favorable response to triptans.
- Always ask if the current headache is similar (or not) to prior headaches the patient may have had.

Acute Back Pain

Causes and Localization

Acute traumatic back pain is, like headache, among the most common symptom for which patients see physicians and is likely a by-product of our walking upright. The vast majority of patients with back pain

Table 2.4 **Quick Exam to Test for Patients with Neck and Back Pain**

Root	Motor	Reflex
C5	Shoulder Abduction and elbow flexion	Biceps
C6	Elbow flexion (while semipronated)	Supinator
C7	Finger and elbow extension	Triceps
C8	Finger flexors	Finger
T1	Hand intrinsic muscles	None
L 3, 4	Extension of knee	Knee jerk
L5	Dorsiflexion of great toe	None
S1	Plantar-flexion of toes	Ankle jerk

have self-limited musculoskeletal conditions that can be treated symptomatically until they resolve on their own. As with headache, the challenge for the clinician is determining which patients harbor serious illnesses and how to develop a diagnostic strategy.

As for localization, physicians must remember that the lesion may be at or above the physical findings. A crisp distinct sensory level is useful at localizing the lesion, but metastases are often multiple, and epidural abscesses can have skip lesions or run along many spinal segments. This becomes important in determining protocol for neuro-imaging tests.

Common causes of neck pain are listed in Table 2.4. The causes of back pain that are potentially life, limb, or cord threatening include:

- Spinal epidural abscess (and vertebral osteomyelitis)
- Metastatic (or primary) tumors of the spine or cord
- Spinal epidural hematoma
- Cord or cauda equina compression due to a central disc herniation (affecting cord or multiple roots)
- Some intra-abdominal and retro-peritoneal processes, such as aortic aneurysm or dissection

Presentation and Evaluations

- The history (in addition to the usual history for a painful condition) should be directed at risk factors for the preceding list.
- Intensity of pain is not an accurate discriminator between severe secondary causes of pain and self-limited mechanical back pain.
- Patients with the aforementioned causes can present with back pain alone in the absence of demonstrable neurological exam

findings. That said, every patient with back pain should have a focused neurological exam of the lower extremities and a test of sensation in the saddle area.
- Always address abnormal vital signs.
- Examine the pulses and abdomen (the physical exam is notoriously inaccurate for aortic aneurysm and dissection.
- Older patients are more likely to have a serious cause, since sciatic is less common in this age group, whereas other illnesses are more common.

Investigations

- For the most part, laboratory testing is not helpful; some recommend using an erythrocyte sedimentation rate to screen for abscess or tumor.
- Plain films are rarely helpful; for serious diagnoses such as spinal epidural abscess (SEA), central disc herniation, or spinal hematoma, they are routinely normal; for tumor, they can be normal (more commonly with lymphoma and less commonly with carcinomas). Furthermore, even when positive for metastases, a MRI will be needed anyway.

- CT scans are much better for trauma and not as sensitive for other problems.
- MRI is the test of choice for all of the serious spine/cord problems already listed. However, MRI is expensive and not universally available. MRI is not needed for typical sciatica patients, whose diagnosis is clinical. Furthermore, many asymptomatic normal individuals with no history of back pain will show disc bulges on MRI. For all these reasons, MRI should be used selectively.
- Consider MRI in the following situations in patients with back pain:
  - Fever, sweats, weight loss, history of IV drug use, prior cancer, HIV, anticoagulant therapy, prior spine surgery
  - Any new neurological signs (other than single root sciatica)
  - Failure of conservative treatment
  - Recent spinal anesthesia
  - Persistent pain that is worse at night
- Note that the timing of the MRI does not always need to be immediate in patients who are neurologically normal. Depending upon the specifics of the situation, planned delay for imaging by hours to days may be indicated.
- Figure 2.1 provides a suggested algorithm for evaluation of non-traumatic neck pain.

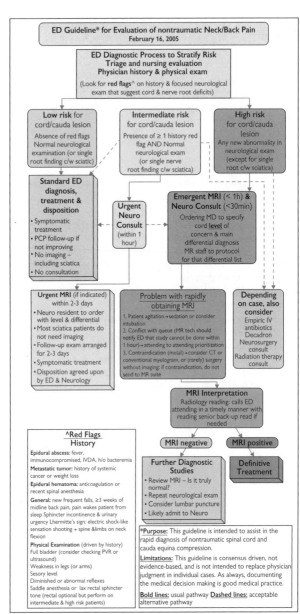

ED Guideline* for Evaluation of nontraumatic Neck/Back Pain
February 16, 2005

ED Diagnostic Process to Stratify Risk
Triage and nursing evaluation
Physician history & physical exam

(Look for **red flags**^ on history & focused neurological exam that suggest cord & nerve root deficits)

Low risk for cord/cauda lesion
Absence of red flags
Normal neurological examination (or single root finding c/w sciatic)

Intermediate risk for cord/cauda lesion
Presence of ≥ 1 history red flag AND Normal neurological exam (or single nerve root finding c/w sciatica)

High risk for cord/cauda lesion
Any new abnormality in neurological exam (except for single root c/w sciatica)

Standard ED diagnosis, treatment & disposition
• Symptomatic treatment
• PCP follow-up if not improving
• No imaging – including sciatica
• No consultation

Urgent Neuro Consult
(within 1 hour)

Emergent MRI (< 1h) & **Neuro Consult** (<30min)
Ordering MD to specify cord **level** of concern & main differential diagnosis
MR staff to protocol for the differential list

Urgent MRI (if indicated) within 2-3 days
• Neuro resident to order with level & differential
• Most sciatica patients do not need imaging
• Follow-up exam arranged for 2-3 days
• Symptomatic treatment
• Disposition agreed upon by ED & Neurology

Problem with rapidly obtaining MRI
1. Patient agitation → sedation or consider intubation
2. Conflict with queue (MR tech should notify ED that study cannot be done within 1 hour) → attending to attending prioritization
3. Contraindication (metal) → consider CT or conventional myelogram, or (rarely) surgery without imaging; if contraindication, do not send to MR suite

Depending on case, also consider
Empiric IV antibiotics
Decadron
Neurosurgery consult
Radiation therapy consult

MRI Interpretation
Radiology reading: calls ED attending in a timely manner with reading senior back-up read if needed

MRI negative

MRI positive

Further Diagnostic Studies
• Review MRI – Is it truly normal?
• Repeat neurological exam
• Consider lumbar puncture
• Likely admit to Neuro

Definitive Treatment

^Red Flags
History

Epidural abscess: fever, immunocompromised, IVDA, h/o bacteremia
Metastatic tumor: history of systemic cancer or weight loss
Epidural hematoma: anticoagulation or recent spinal anesthesia
General: new frequent falls, ≥3 weeks of midline back pain, pain wakes patient from sleep Sphincter incontinence & urinary urgency Lhermitte's sign: electric shock-like sensation shooting → spine &limbs on neck flexion
Physical Examination (driven by history)
Full bladder (consider checking PVR or ultrasound)
Weakness in legs (or arms)
Sesory level
Diminished or abnormal reflexes
Saddle anesthesia or lax rectal sphincter tone (rectal optional but perform on intermediate & high risk patients)

*Purpose: This guideline is intended to assist in the rapid diagnosis of nontraumatic spinal cord and cauda equina compression.

Limitations: This guideline is consensus driven, not evidence-based, and is not intended to replace physician judgment in individual cases. As always, documenting the medical decision making is good medical practice.

Bold lines: usual pathway **Dashed lines:** acceptable alternative pathway

Figure 2.1 Suggested algorithm for evaluation of non-traumatic neck pain.

Clinical Pearls

- Patients with serious disease may have normal neurological exams at the time of initial presentation.
- Fever is absent in half of cases of patients with SEA.
- Spinal metastases can be the presenting symptom of cancer. Therefore, not every patient will have a known history of cancer.
- Classic presentations are rarely the most common ones.
- Depending on which roots are involved, cauda equina lesions my present with predominant bowel or bladder symptoms in the absence of more distal weakness.

Diplopia

Causes and Localization

- Chapter 8 on Cranial Neuropathy discusses the various cranial nerve lesions (both individual and combined) that cause diplopia. The reader is referred to that section for localization and evaluation.
- Diplopia can be characterized as monocular or binocular and traumatic or nontraumatic.
- Traumatic diplopia is generally caused by a fracture of the orbit, with entrapment of an extra-ocular muscle or contusion of a cranial nerve or extra-ocular muscle.

Presentation

- On the surface, it would seem that all patients with diplopia would present with a sudden onset, since they either see more than one image or not. However, this is not always the case. If the separation of the two images is slight, a patient might only complain of blurred vision.
- Patients with monocular diplopia almost always have an ophthalmologic cause; these include refractive errors as well as lid, corneal, and retinal pathology.
- Patients with horizontal diplopia usually have a sixth nerve palsy.

Investigations

- See Figure 2.2 for an algorithmic approach to the evaluation of patients with diplopia.
- In patients with traumatic diplopia, thin-cut orbital CT is the initial test of choice.
- In patients with monocular diplopia, a very thorough eye exam is important. Ophthalmologic consultation ought to be performed in most cases.

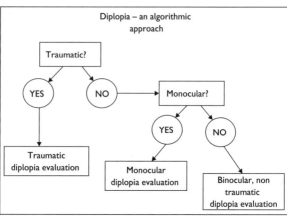

Figure 2.2 Suggested algorithm for evaluation of diplopia.

- Patients with nontraumatic binocular diplopia require enough of a work-up to identify the lesion, since many of the causes require specific therapy. Neurological consultation is recommended in most cases.

Clinical Pearls

- Sixth nerve palsy has little localizing value; its long course makes it very sensitive to meningeal inflammation and elevations (and severe decreases) in ICP. Sixth nerve palsy is the most common cranial neuropathy causing diplopia.
- Patients with diplopia whose image separation is slight may complain not of double vision but of blurred vision.
- Binocular diplopia resolves with covering of either eye, whereas monocular diplopia resolves only with covering the affected eye.
- Distinguish between pupil-involving versus pupil-sparing third nerve palsy.
- Consider testing for thyroid disease in patients with binocular nontraumatic diplopia.
- Patients with fourth nerve palsy usually tilt their head away from the side of the lesion.

Dizziness and Vertigo

Causes and Localization

One of the most difficult diagnostic problems in clinical medicine is the dizzy patient. As with any pure sensory symptom, patients can have great difficulty describing their symptoms when they feel dizzy

Table 2.5	**Categorization of Dizziness by Symptom Quality**			
	Vertigo	**Near-syncope**	**Disequilibrium**	**Other**
Definition	Illusory sense of motion, usually felt in the head	Sensation of near faint, "blacking out" or "graying out", usually felt in the head	Feeling gait unsteadiness, usually felt in the body	Does not fit into other boxes
Suggested diagnoses	Vestibular or posterior circulation problems	Cardiovascular issues	Combination of factors that can include multiple minor neurological issues (e.g., neuropathy, poor vision or hearing, etc), poly-pharmacy & others	Often psychiatric disorders

*In this scheme, ask, "What do you mean dizzy?" Wait for the patient to answer with a response that puts them into one of the four categories above. See text for further discussion of its history and limitations.

and the language of dizziness is imperfect at best. The cornerstone of any diagnosis—the history—is more difficult to pin down in these patients. Finally, the differential diagnosis of unselected patients who complain of dizziness is vast.

The traditional approach to diagnosing the dizzy patient is to use nondirected questions in order to place the patient into one of four pathophysiologic categories (see Table 2.5). These questions are, "What do you mean dizzy?" or "Can you tell me how you feel without using the word *dizzy*?" This diagnostic framework was derived from work done in the 1970s and involved patients who were ultimately referred to ENT- or neurology-run dizziness clinics. This population is obviously quite different from the acute, nonselected group of dizzy patients that present acutely to an ED. This latter population of patients includes those with systemic infections, volume depletion, cardiac and gastrointestinal problems, and others. They are not so easily categorized using the traditional system.

Newer research on this unselected group shows that patients frequently change their answers to the preceding questions when asked the same question minutes later. As well, a patient's use of the word *vertigo* or *lightheaded* (or any of the other words that patients might use) is not predictive of a cause. Furthermore, many patients select more than one category of dizziness. Finally, new research indicates that patients are more accurate in answering questions about the duration and triggers of their dizzy symptoms. There are essentially three categories in this pathophysiologic system, based on timing and triggers

Table 2.6 **Categorization of Dizziness by Timing and Triggers***

Pattern 1: Prolonged continuous dizziness

Starts acutely and lasts days to weeks.

Pattern 2: Episodes of spontaneous dizziness

Spontaneous episodes that come acutely and usually last minutes to hours. They are not precipitated by changes in head position.

Pattern 3: Episodes of positional dizziness

*In this scheme, the timing and triggers, which research shows is more accurately reported, drives the differential diagnosis and diagnostic work-up.

(see Table 2.6). It is important to emphasize that a patient's use of the word *vertigo*, *lightheaded*, or of phrases like "I feel like I'm going to faint" (or any other) is less important than the timing of the symptoms.

In the timing and triggers approach, the temporal patterns suggest a differential diagnosis. The major differential diagnosis for the first pattern is cerebellar infarction and vestibular neuritis. The major differential diagnosis for the second pattern is transient ischemic attack (TIA) versus migraine-related dizziness. The large majority of patients with the third pattern have benign paroxysmal positional vertigo (BPPV). It is important to note that some patients with BPPV will have a more continuous fear or anxiety about becoming vertiginous and thus describe their symptoms as constant and not episodic. It is also important to know that patients who have vestibular neuritis or a cerebellar mass or stroke will also have worsening symptoms with head movement.

Understanding these facts, physicians can and must take a very careful history designed to tease out these facts in order to place the patient into the correct temporal pattern.

In addition to these two different ways of thinking about acutely dizzy patients, there is another diagnostic factor that the physician must consider—is the underlying cause a CNS problem or is it a peripheral vestibular problem? Importantly, a central cause is not necessarily life-threatening (e.g., migrainous vertigo), but it is still useful to think of neurological conditions in this way.

With one exception, patients who present with simultaneous onset of both diminished hearing and vertigo generally have a peripheral problem. This is due to the fact that the end-organs (the cochlea and the labyrinth) are co-located peripherally. The exception is infarction in the territory of the anterior inferior cerebellar artery, which supplies the cochlea via the internal auditory artery. Vertigo with other cranial nerve or long tract signs or symptoms suggests a brainstem lesion, and vertigo with abnormal cerebellar function suggests a cerebellar problem. Table 2.7 summarizes the features that distinguish between peripheral and central vertigo.

Test	Peripheral	Central
Quality of nystagmus	Unidirectional horizontalTorsional (in Dix-Hallpike)	Direction-changing Pure vertical
Head thrust maneuver	Positive test (presence of a corrective saccade)	Negative test
Dix-Hallpike maneuver	Positive	Negative (although changes in position may worsen any vertigo to some extent)
Gait	Unsteady but usually able to walk	May be unable to walk or stand
Other neurological findings on exam	Absent (with the possible exception of acute hearing loss)	Usually present if tested for

Table 2.7 Methods to Distinguish Central Vertigo from Peripheral

Presentation

- Because the differential diagnosis of dizziness is vast, physicians must use elements of the history and physical examination to decide what work-up to pursue. The preceding discussion notwithstanding, there are no prospectively collected data that argue for an algorithmic evaluation (or history) that works in all patients. Flesh out the history in terms of the following aspects:
  - When did the dizziness start?
  - Has it been constant or intermittent?
  - If intermittent, what are the triggers that seem to make it worse?
  - Are there other components of the chief complaint (pain, fluid loss, fever, shortness of breath (SOB), other neurological symptoms, etc)?
  - How does the patient describe their dizziness?
  - Have there been any recent medication changes?
- The physical examination starts with evaluation of the vital signs, which may suggest an etiology or group of etiologies.
- With the understanding that a complete neurological exam should be done, it is particularly important to perform a careful examination of cerebellar functions. Eye movements can be very useful in characterizing a patient's dizziness and these could be omitted in a cursory exam that focuses on lateralizing motor findings.

- The examination should also include watching the patient walk, unless there is some other obvious reason not to do this (e.g., clear-cut volume depletion or myocardial ischemia).

Investigations

- As was already mentioned, there is no prospective study to guide how these patients ought to be evaluated and to what extent the various diagnostic schemes mentioned earlier are useful. There is no clinical decision rule on which patients benefit from advanced diagnostic imaging.
- There is a wide range of possible tests that could be appropriate for an acutely dizzy patient, because the differential diagnosis is vast.
- Abnormal vital signs (including the SaO2) need to be addressed carefully; the work-up for many of these issues is beyond the scope of this book. For example, a fever suggests a systemic infection (pneumonia, urosepsis, etc.), and testing for those conditions should be undertaken. Tachycardia and/or hypotension suggest another set of possibilities: sepsis, volume depletion, and acute blood loss, etc. The important point is to pay careful attention to the vital signs as they usually offer clues to the ultimate diagnosis.
- Patients with brief episodes of positional dizziness should have a Dix-Hallpike maneuver performed, which tests the posterior semi-circular canal. This accounts for ~ 85 percent of cases of BPPV.
- An electrocardiogram may be useful in cases in which the cause is not obvious from the history and physical examination.

Clinical Pearls

- As many as 10 percent of patients with ischemic cerebellar stroke present with symptoms that mimic an acute peripheral vestibular syndrome.
- The head thrust maneuver is an easy-to-perform bedside test to distinguish cerebellar infarction from acute vestibular neuritis.
- Know your nystagmus (see Table 2.8).
- Have every dizzy patient walk unless there is an obvious diagnosis that precludes the need for gait testing.
- Cranial CT is notoriously insensitive for posterior circulation ischemia and infarction—a normal CT does not exclude a cerebellar or brainstem stroke.
- Explain all abnormal vital signs.

Table 2.8 Interpretation of Nystagmus*

Finding – type of nystagmus	Interpretation	Comments
Unilateral horizontal nystagmus	Usually found in a peripheral cause of vertigo	Watch carefully to other side; sometimes there will be nystagmus to both sides, but the direction of the fast phase is the same
Direction-changing nystagmus	In "*nonpositional*" vertigo, this finding means a central cause	Note that direction changing nystagmus can be found in some forms of "*positional*" vertigo - BPPV
Vertical nystagmus	This usually indicates a central vertigo	
Torsional nystagmus	Can be central or peripheral	This is common with typical BPPV
End-gaze nystagmus	Physiologic	Note that many normal people will have a few beats of horizontal nystagmus on far end gaze

*The interpretation of nystagmus must be made in the context of the pattern of vertigo; for example, the same finding may indicated a central cause of vertigo in a patient with a prolonged episode of vertigo but something entirely different in someone with positional episodes of vertigo.
Abbreviations: BPPV = benign paroxysmal positional vertigo

- Most patients with BPPV and a positive Dix-Hallpike can be treated with an Epley (canal repositioning) maneuver and do not need diagnostic testing or medications.
- Remember that patients whose histories suggest BPPV, but whose Dix-Hallpike test is negative, may have BPPV of the horizontal semicircular canals (and not the posterior canal, which is tested in the Dix-Hallpike).

Speech Difficulties

It is important when evaluating patients with speech difficulties to distinguish aphasia from dysarthria.

- Aphasia refers to loss or impairment of language processing.

Table 2.9 **Causes of Mutism**
Psychiatric disorders
Hyperacute/acute phase of aphasia
Akinetic mutism due to bilateral frontal lesions
Locked-in syndrome
Advanced lower motor neuron disease, such as Guillain-Barré syndrome

- Dysarthria, on the other hand, is a motor speech disorder in which speech articulation is impaired. However, other language functions such as reading, writing, and comprehension are unaffected.

Causes and Localization

- Stroke involving the perisylvian language cortex is the most common cause of aphasia. However, any other focal lesion affecting the language areas, such as neoplasms or infections (abscess or HSV encephalitis) can also cause aphasia.
- Aphasia can occasionally result from focal lesions (mostly stroke) confined to subcortical structures strongly interconnected with language cortices. These include lesions involving the dominant anterolateral thalamus or striatocapsular lesions involving the dominant putamen, dorsolateral part of the caudate, anterior limb of the internal capsule, and rostral periventricular white matter.
  - Patients with acute-onset aphasia may be mute (total cessation of verbal output) for the first few days. See Table 2.9.
- Diffuse lesions producing widespread neuronal dysfunction, such as traumatic brain injury or degenerative conditions (dementia) can also cause aphasia.
- Dysarthria is poorly localizing. Any lesion that affects respiration (lungs, chest wall, or diaphragm), phonation (larynx), articulation (lips, teeth, tongue), resonance (pharynx), or prosody can produce dysarthric speech.
- Dysarthria does not always indicate a brain lesion, but when due to a central cause these lesions can be unilateral or bilateral; cortical or subcortical; or affecting the brainstem, cranial nerves, or cerebellum. See Table 2.10.

Presentation and Evaluation

- The following systematic approach is recommended when evaluating patients with speech difficulty:
  - Determine the nature of the speech abnormality, that is, aphasia vs. dysarthria vs. mutism.

Table 2.10 **Causes of Dysarthria**	
Acute onset	• Drugs (e.g., Alcohol) • Stroke • Encephalitis (e.g., HSV)
Subacute onset	• Infections • Neoplasm • Metabolic disturbance • Drugs (e.g., anti-convulsants)
Chronic (progressive)	• Multiple sclerosis • Extrapyramidal disease (e.g., Parkinson's) • Motor neuron disease • Dementia

- Determine the onset (acute vs. subacute/chronic) and the rate of progression of symptoms.
  - Slowly progressive isolated language impairment in older patients with signs of cognitive decline is suggestive of a dementing illness, such as frontotemporal dementia or Alzheimer's disease.
  - Acute onset suggests a stroke or metabolic disturbance, in particular hypoglycemia.
  - Subacute onset may suggest a neoplastic or infectious cause.
- Determine the presence of other associated symptoms and signs, such as hemiparesis, visual field abnormalities, diplopia, cognitive difficulties, shortness of breath, etc.
- In order to distinguish language impairment from purely motor deficits (dysarthria), one needs to assess for all of the following language components:
  - Fluency, which refers to the rate, quantity, and ease of speech production. In nonfluent speech, verbal output is reduced and effortful, and phrase length is short.
    - Nonfluency, in the absence of a toxic-metabolic abnormality, often indicates involvement of the frontal language regions.
    - Paraphasic errors, which refer to substitution of incorrect words for intended words (e.g., *orange* for *apple*) or when a part of a word is misspoken (e.g., *mapple* for *apple*) are common in aphasics and can occur with lesions anywhere within the language regions.
  - Comprehension, which refers to the ability to understand spoken language and to follow verbal commands.
    - Impairment of comprehension often indicates damage to the temporoparietal language region.

- It is important to point out that patients with comprehension difficulties are often mislabeled as confused, especially when other components of language function are not fully assessed.
- Repetition, which refers to the ability to repeat spoken phrases.
  - Impaired repetition often indicates involvement of the language cortices.
  - **Repetition is almost always intact in patients with subcortical aphasia. Therefore, it can be an important localizing sign.**
- Naming: Word-finding is always impaired in patients with aphasia. Occasionally, aphasics talk around the words that they fail to retrieve by providing descriptions to convey the meanings of the words (circumlocutions).
- Reading and writing: Reading and writing impairments parallel oral language comprehension and production deficits in aphasic patients. See Table 2.11.
- Although dysarthric speech may be seen in patients with Broca's aphasia, most patients with dysarthria are not aphasic.
- Several types (presentations) of nonaphasic dysarthria may be distinguished and are summarized in Table 2.12. They can be distinguished from aphasic dysarthria by demonstrating that other language functions, in particular writing, are intact.
- Two distinct syndromes are worth mentioning:
  - Alexia without agraphia, where patient's ability to read is severely impaired despite preserved speech, comprehension, repetition, and writing. Interestingly, patients can write but cannot read their own writing. A right homonymous hemianopia and color anomia are often present, since the causative lesion is usually in the left occipital lobe and splenium of the corpus callosum.
  - Pure word deafness: These patients resemble those with Wernicke's aphasia. However, unlike Wernicke's aphasia, comprehension of written material is intact and writing is normal. The causative lesions are usually in the superior temporal cortices.

Investigations

- Laboratory studies including complete blood cell count, serum glucose, urine analysis, and toxicology screen will identify most potential infectious and metabolic causes of speech difficulties.
- Brain neuroimaging (CT scan or preferably MRI) will identify most focal brain lesions.
- Electromyography may be required to diagnose neuromuscular disorders causing dysarthria.

Table 2.11 Clinical features of various aphasic syndromes					
Clinical syndrome	Repetition	Fluency	Comprehension	Hemiparesis	Visual field defect
Broca's	Poor	Poor	Good	Common	Rare
Wernicke's	Poor	Good	Poor	Rare	Common
Global	Poor	Poor	Poor	Common	Common
TC motor	Intact	Poor	Good	Variable	Rare
TC sensory	Intact	Good	Poor	Variable	Common
Mixed TC	Intact	Poor	Poor	Common	Common
Thalamic	Intact	Good	Poor	Rare	Variable
Striatocapsular	Intact	Variable	Good	Common	Rare

Type	Causes	Localization	Distinctive Features
Paretic (flaccid)	• Bulbar palsy • Myopathy • Neuromuscular junction disorders	Lower motor neuron lesion	Low-pitched, nasal voice
Spastic	• Pseudibulbar palsy due to bilateral lesions	Upper motor neuron lesion	Slow and monotonic speech
Ataxic	• Cerebellar lesion • Multiple sclerosis	Cerebellur lesions	Jerky and dysrhythmic speech with excessive stress
Extrapyramidal; • Hypokinetic • Hyperkinetic	Parkinson's disease Chorea	Extrapyramidal system	Monopitch and monotone Highly variable with hypernasality
Mixed	• Multiple sclerosis • Amyotrophic lateral sclerosis	Multiple motor system involvement	Variable and mixed pattern

Table 2.12 **Types of Dysarthria**

- Lumbar puncture may be indicated in cases in which there is suspicion for HSV encephalitis.
- Electroencephalogram may be indicated in patients with isolated stereotyped aphasia to rule out a focal epileptic focus.

Acute Visual Changes

The causes and localization of lesions in patients who complain of visual changes depend on:

- Whether one (monocular) or both (binocular) eyes are affected.
- The nature of the visual changes and whether it is partial vs. complete in cases of visual loss.
- The onset and course of the visual changes—abrupt vs. gradual.
- The presence or absence of associated symptoms, such as eye pain, headaches, etc.
- Age of the patient.

Causes and Localization

- The unique organization of the visual pathways from the retina to the visual cortex allows accurate localization of the lesion based on physical examination.
- Visual acuity is often preserved in patients with visual loss due to lesions of the visual cortices.
- There are several causes for acute transient monocular blindness (TMB):
  - The most common cause of TMB is retinal embolism.
  - The following are causes of acute visual loss:
    - Local intra-ocular pathology, such as glaucoma, drusen, papilledema, anterior ischemic optic neuropathy.
    - Intermittent vascular compression from intra-orbital lesions such as meningioma.
    - Retinal embolization leading to central or branch retinal artery occlusion. Causes include:
      - Cardioembolism
      - Aortic atherosclerosis
      - Carotid disease
      - Hematological disorders such as polycythemia
    - Vasospasm as seen in migraine and hypertensive crisis.
  - The causes for subacute monocular visual loss tend to be age dependent.
    - Optic neuritis is the most common cause in younger patients. It is often painful and the pain is worse with eye movements.
    - Anterior ischemic optic neuropathy (AION) is the most common cause in elderly patients over 60 years of age. There are two forms of AION:
      - Nonarteritic: usually painless.
      - Arteritic: due to temporal arteritis. Associated symptoms of headaches, tenderness of the scalp, shoulder pains, weight loss, and jaw claudication are often present.
    - Chronic progressive monocular visual loss usually indicates chronic optic nerve compression from chronic papilledema, glaucoma, or retro-orbital tumor.
- Some causes of acute binocular visual loss include:
  - Bilateral optic disk or nerve diseases. This is rare.
  - Vasospasm due to migraine or contrast material following arterial angiography.
  - Brain tumors causing increased ICP, especially those involving the frontal lobe or olfactory groove meningioma.
  - Bilateral occipital or parieto-occipital lesions.
  - Trauma leading to chiasmal tear.

- Pituitary apoplexy.
  - The most common cause of abrupt binocular visual loss is a frontal tumor causing monocular visual loss and optic atrophy in one eye and papilledema in the other eye.
  - It is not uncommon that patients presenting with abrupt binocular visual loss may have not noticed visual loss in the first eye, and that the loss of vision in the "good" eye suddenly made them realize that they could no longer see. This can be seen in bilateral optic disk diseases, such as optic neuritis or optic neuropathy.
  - Patients with chiasmal lesions may present with binocular visual loss. For example:
    - Pituitary tumors may cause superior bitemporal visual loss.
    - Anterior cerebral artery aneurysm or craniopharyngioma may cause inferior bitemporal visual loss.
  - Bilateral visual loss may be the result of homonymous hemianopia caused by lesions involving the optic tract, lateral geniculate nucleus of the thalamus, tracts from the geniculate nucleus to the visual cortex, or the occipital cotex.
    - Isolated dense hemianopia, without other symptoms, is usually seen with involvement of the optic tracts or the occipital cortex
    - Lesions between the optic tract and visual cortex are often associated with other symptoms and signs such as hemiparesis, sensory loss, neglect, or aphasia.

Presentation and Evaluation

- The bedside evaluation of patients with visual complaints should include:
  - Assessment of visual acuity. Visual acuity should be within normal in patients with pure visual field loss (hemianopia)
  - Assessment of visual field by confrontation method.
  - Color vision testing (using Ishihara's color plates), especially in patients with suspected optic nerve damage.
  - Pupillary testing: This should include swinging the light from eye to eye to look for an afferent pupillary defect. This would imply optic nerve damage and consists of a less brisk constriction of the pupil in the affected eye or even its dilatation in response to light compared to the unaffected eye/pupil.
  - Funduscopic examination: to assess for the presence of disk pallor, ocular changes, papilledema, or cholesterol emboli (Hollenhorst plaque).
- Acute transient visual loss should be differentiated from visual obscuration, where the visual symptoms only last for seconds and can be monocular or binocular. These are often seen with glaucoma, papilledema, and disk drusen.

- It is important to inquire about the descriptive details and nature of the patient's complaint of visual loss, because the term may be used to describe other visual changes.
  - Painful visual loss suggests the possibility of glaucoma, temporal arteritis, pseudotumor cerebri, or other causes of increased ICP, optic neuritis, or pituitary apoplexy
- The following diagnoses should always be kept in mind when evaluating patients with acute visual loss, because early recognition and treatment can significantly improve outcome:
  - Ischemic optic neuropathy due to temporal arteritis
  - Acute glaucoma
  - Central retinal artery occlusion
  - Pseudotumor cerebri (benign intracranial hypertension)
  - Retrobulbar mass lesion
  - Pituitary apoplexy
- The following conditions are worth mentioning:
  - Pituitary apoplexy is a true emergency. It occurs due to hemorrhage into the pituitary gland, often into a previously undiagnosed adenoma. Presenting features include: headache; agitation; stiff neck; fever; CN III, IV, and VI palsies, resulting in disturbances of ocular motility; and acute unilateral or bilateral visual loss. Diagnosis requires a high degree of suspicion and can be confirmed with MRI or CT scan, the former being more sensitive.
  - Anton's syndrome, in which patients develop complete visual loss due to bilateral infarctions of the occipital lobes. A characteristic feature is that these patients tend to deny blindness and confabulate when asked to name objects.
  - Balint's syndrome: This is caused by bilateral damage, mostly stroke, to the parieto-occipital regions. Patients loose their ability to perceive more than one object at a time, to voluntarily guide eye movements or change to a new location of visual fixation, or to coordinate eye movements. As a result, they present with vague bilateral visual complaints.
- The presence of positive visual symptoms, such as seeing zigzag lines, bright light or glimmer, flashes or sparkles, should raise the possibility of retinal detachment; migraine aura, especially if the symptoms gradually build up and move from the center to the periphery; or occipital seizures, especially in patients with known occipital lesions.

Investigations

- Laboratory studies, including complete blood cell count, erythrocyte sedimentation rate, and c-reactive protein, to assess for temporal arteritis.
- Detailed funduscopic examination.

- Brain neuroimaging (CT scan or preferably MRI) will identify most focal brain lesions.
- Lumbar puncture may be indicated in cases in which there is suspicion for elevated ICP (assuming no contraindications on brain imaging) or demyelination.
- Visual evoked responses may be indicated in patients with suspected optic neuritis.
- Hypercoagulable studies; an echocardiogram; and extracranial ultrasound, CTA or MRA; may be indicated in patients with TMB.

Acute Hearing Loss

Hearing loss can be conductive or sensorineural.
- Conductive hearing loss occurs when the sound cannot reach the cochlea due to abnormalities of the ear canal, the tympanic membrane, or the middle ear ossicles.
- Sensorineural hearing loss results from lesions involving the cochlea or CN VIII.

Causes

There are several causes for sudden and abrupt hearing loss. These are summarized in Table 2.13.
- The most common causes of conductive hearing loss are trauma or infections.
- Sensorineural hearing loss may be hereditary.

Table 2.13 Causes of Sudden Hearing Loss
Idiopathic
Trauma: (1) head injury with or without fracture or hemorrhage involving the cochlea; (2) Barotrauma caused by large ambient pressure changes or strenuous physical activities: can induce a perilymphatic fistula between the middle and inner ear.
Infections: mumps and measles, varicella, adenoviruses, Epstein-Barr virus, syphilis, cytomegalovirus, HSV, and other occult viral or bacterial infections.
Vascular disorders: involving the terminal branch of the anterior inferior cerebellar artery cause ischemia of the eighth cranial nerve, especially in diabetics.
Hematological conditions: Waldenström's macroglobulinemia, sickle cell disease, and leukemia.
Ototoxic drugs: such as aminoglycosides.

- Unilateral progressive hearing loss should raise suspicion for an underlying acoustic neuroma.
  - Bilateral acoustic neuromas may be seen in patients with neurofibromatosis type II.
- The following condition is worth mentioning:
  - Perilymphatic fistula is an abnormal opening between the air-filled middle ear and the fluid-filled inner ear. Head trauma and barotraumas are the most common causes, but it may also result from chronic ear infections (cholesteatomas). Symptoms include hearing loss, dizziness, vertigo, imbalance, motion intolerance, nausea, and vomiting. Pressure sensitivity is a common and characteristic symptom. When a fistula is present, changes in middle ear pressure may directly affect the inner ear, stimulating the balance and/or hearing structures and causing typical symptoms. Thus, patients often report worsening symptoms with coughing, sneezing, and with exertion and activity.
    - Acute cochlear neuritis, is similar in presumed pathophysiology to Bell's palsy, but involves the cochlear component of the eighth nerve. The hearing loss comes on over hours, is sometimes associated with aural fullness and, in some cases, there is partial hearing loss associated with abnormal harsh or distorted sounds. Weber test (see Presentation and Evaluation section that follows) will localize away from the lesion. Although the data for steroid use are limited, most authorities recommend a course of steroids to minimize permanent hearing loss.

Presentation and Evaluation

- Evaluation should begin with detailed history of medications, co-morbid conditions and presenting symptoms, and otologic examination of the external ear canal and the tympanic membrane.
  - Hearing loss may range in severity from mild to profound, and it may occur alone or in association with other symptoms, such as vertigo, tinnitus, nausea, or vomiting.
  - Associated ear pain or discharge from the ear often points to an infectious cause.
  - The presence of associated nystagmus, tinnitus, and vertigo may be indicative of a vascular cause, such as an anterior inferior cerebellar artery territory infarct or a perilymphatic fistula.
  - History of stereotyped recurrent episodes of tinnitus, hearing loss, and dizziness suggests Meniere's disease.

- Tuning fork tests are important bedside tests to differentiate conductive from sensoineural hearing loss.
  - Weber's test: The tuning fork is placed on the middle of the forehead equidistant from the patient's ears. The patient is asked to report in which ear the sound is heard louder.
    - In normal individuals and in those with bilateral symmetrical hearing loss, the sound is heard equally loud in both ears (no lateralization).
    - A patient with a unilateral conductive hearing loss would hear the tuning fork loudest in the affected ear.
    - A patient with a unilateral sensorineural hearing loss would hear the sound loudest in the unaffected ear.
  - Rinne's test: This is performed by alternating the placement of the tuning fork firmly on the mastoid bone (to assess bone conduction) and opposite the corresponding external auditory meatus (to assess air conduction), and asking the patient to compare the loudness of the fork in these locations.
    - In normal individuals, air conduction lasts twice as long as bone conduction.
    - A patient with conductive hearing loss will hear the fork sound longer by bone conduction, while a patient with sensorineural loss will hear the fork longer by air conduction.
  - Rinne's and Weber's tests can be complimentary:
    - If the Rinne's test shows that air conduction is greater than bone conduction in both ears and the Weber's test lateralizes to a particular ear, then there is sensorineural hearing loss in the opposite (weaker) ear.
    - Conductive hearing loss is confirmed in the weaker ear if bone conduction is greater than air conduction and the Weber's test lateralizes to that side.
    - Combined hearing loss is likely if the Weber's test lateralizes to the stronger ear and bone conduction is greater than air conduction in the weaker ear.

Investigations

- Formal audiologic evaluation and audiogram is recommended in almost all patients
- Laboratory studies including complete blood cell count, erythrocyte sedimentation rate, and rapid plasma regain (RPR).
- Brain MRI may be required in cases in which a vascular cause or acoustic neuroma is suspected.
- Tympanometry, electronystagmography (ENG), and a CT scan of the temporal bone may be required if a perilymphatic fistula is suspected.

Acute Weakness

When patients report weakness, it is important to distinguish generalized fatigue from true muscle weakness. The causes of acute weakness are detailed later in chapter 6.

The first step in evaluating patients with confirmed acute muscle weakness is to determine if it is due to an upper or motor neuron lesion.

- The presence of upper motor neuron signs such as hyperreflexia, hemisensory loss, upgoing toes, or cranial nerve abnormalities provide clues to a central cause.
  - The presence of cranial nerve abnormalities points to a brain lesion.
  - The presence of a sensory level points to a spinal cord lesion.
- The distribution of weakness provides important clues to the cause:
  - Symmetrical proximal muscle weakness involving the deltoids, biceps, or thigh muscles suggests a neuromuscular cause, such as Guillain-Barre syndrome or a myopathic process.
  - Symmetric distal muscle weakness is more likely to be related to a neuropathic process.
  - Asymmetric muscle weakness could be caused by a mononeuropathy, plexopathy, or a central process, that is, brain or spinal cord lesions.

Appropriate diagnostic tests and investigations depend on the suspected localization and etiology of the lesion.

- Brain imaging or MRI of the spine is indicated if an upper motor neuron lesion is suspected.
  - If the whole spine is not imaged, spine imaging should include all spinal cord levels above the sensory level detected on examination.
- Laboratory tests including CBC, erythrocyte sedimentation rate (ESR), serum electrolytes (especially potassium), thyroid stimulating hormone (TSH), and creatine phosphokinase (CPK) should be obtained in patients with suspected myopathy; ESR, TSH, Lyme serology, glycosylated hemoglobin (A1C), and protein electrophoresis should be evaluated in patients with neuropathy
- Lumbar puncture may be indicated in suspected Guillain-Barre syndrome or demyelinating lesions.
- Electromyography (EMG), nerve conduction study (NCS), and muscle or nerve biopsies may be required in some cases.

Suggested Reading

Clark LW. Communication disorders: what to look for, and when to refer. *Geriatrics.* 1994;49(6):51–55.

Comer RM, et al. Causes and outcomes for patients presenting with diplopia to an eye casualty department. *Eye* 2007;2:413–416.

Edlow JA, et al. Update on subarachnoid hemorrhage for emergency physicians. *J Emerg Med.* 2008;34:237–251.

Edlow JA, et al. Diagnosis and initial management of cerebellar infarction. *Lancet Neurology.* 2008;7:951–964.

Jordan LC, Hillis AE. Disorders of speech and language: aphasia, apraxia and dysarthria. *Curr Opin Neurol.* 2006;19(6):580–585.

Kent RD. Research on speech motor control and its disorders: a review and prospective. *J Commun Disord.* 2000;33(5):391–427.

Koes BW, et al. Diagnosis and treatment of low back pain. *BMJ* 2009;332:1430–1434.

Lavy C, et al. Cauda equina syndrome. *BMJ* 2009;338:881–884.

Luneau K, Newman NJ, Biousse V. Ischemic optic neuropathies. *Neurologist,* 2008;14(6):341–354.

Perkin GD. Neuro-ophthalmologic syndrome for neurologists. *J Neurology Neurosurgery Psychiatry* 2004;75:20–23.

Rauch S. Idiopathic sudden sensorineural hearing loss. *N Engl J Med.* 2008;359:833–840.

Taylor D, Lewis S. Delirium. *J Neurol Neurosurg Psychiatry.* 1993;56(7):742–751.

Vortmann M, Schneider JI. Acute monocular visual loss. *Emerg Med Clin North Am.* 2008;26(1):73–96.

Young GB. Coma. *Ann N Y Acad Sci.* 2008;1157:32–47.

Zadeh MH, Storper IS, Spitzer JB. Diagnosis and treatment of sudden-onset sensorineural hearing loss: a study of 51 patients. *Otolaryngol Head Neck Surg.* 2003;128(1):92–98.

Chapter 3
Cerebral Ischemia

Radoslav Raychev, Sidney Starkman, and
David S. Liebeskind

Introduction

Among all neurological disorders, ischemic stroke is the most common reason for emergency room visits. Over the past two decades, there has been tremendous progress in the approach to treatment of the acute ischemic stroke. Physicians from all backgrounds have realized that brain tissue can be salvaged if patients are evaluated in a timely manner and managed appropriately. In this chapter, we will review the basic principles of pathophysiology, diagnosis, and treatment of ischemic stroke, focusing on the emergent evaluation and rapid therapeutic interventions.

Pathophysiology of Brain Ischemia

Cerebral ischemia results from deprivation of critical nutrient blood flow to brain tissue most commonly from limited arterial antegrade flow, which can be due either to flow-limiting stenosis or complete arterial occlusion. The reduction of regional cerebral blood flow (CBF) leads to disruption of this ionic homeostasis across the cellular membrane and depolarization, with massive influx of calcium into the intracellular space, accumulation of lactic acid, and mitochondrial damage with subsequent release of excitotoxic and inflammatory neurotransmitters, ultimately resulting in cytotoxic edema and cellular death.

Ischemic Core and Ischemic Penumbra

The concept of ischemic core and ischemic penumbra is based on the compartmental distribution of the hypoperfused brain into three distinct zones:

- Ischemic core (CBF 7–12 ml/100 mg/min)—an area of irreversibly damaged brain tissue.
- Ischemic penumbra (CBF 7–22 ml/100 g/min)—an area of hypoperfused and functionally impaired, but still viable brain tissue.
- Benign oligemia (CBF 20 ml/100 g/min–40 ml/100 g/min)—an area of hypoperfused, but functionally intact brain tissue, which is not at risk for infarction.

The volume of these ischemic zones depends mainly on the extent and the duration of hypoperfusion, but is also influenced by a multitude of factors, including the site of vessel occlusion, collateral flow, and other hemodynamic and metabolic factors. The compartmentalization of hypoperfused brain tissue is not absolute and there is substantial degree of overlap. Dynamic changes can lead to incorporation of the oligemic tissue into the ischemic penumbra and into

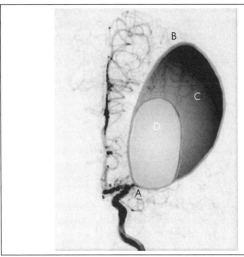

Figure 3.1 Angiographic representation of acute cerebral ischemia. (a) arterial occlusion, (b) region of benign oligemia, (c) penumbra, and (d) ischemic core.

infarction. Conversely, timely delivery of blood flow into the hypoperfused area can result in complete resolution of the ischemic penumbra and reversal to normal. This concept of salvageable ischemic penumbra is the main target of therapeutic interventions in acute ischemic stroke (Figure 3.1).

The principal strategy for acute intervention is aimed at arterial recanalization to achieve effective reperfusion. Several investigators have used diffusion/perfusion MRI to demonstrate the presence of penumbral tissue, where diffusion abnormalities represent bioenergetic compromise and the perfusion abnormalities reflect hemodynamic compromise. Thus, the concept of mismatch between functional and structural changes with evolving ischemia has been introduced.

Mechanisms of Ischemic Stroke

There are two key mechanisms that may culminate in cerebral ischemia:

- Thromboembolism, compromising the arterial lumen, which can occur either as a result of in-situ thrombosis or embolism from a proximal source, leading to abrupt cessation of flow, downstream from the compromised vessel.

• Hemodynamic failure, which can occur either as a result of failure of collateral flow in acute arterial occlusion or rarely in conditions associated with systemic hypotension and inadequate cerebral perfusion.

Thromboembolism and hypoperfusion often coexist and equally contribute to the final outcome in ischemic stroke. The status of the occluded artery has become the major target of acute stroke interventions. However, cerebral hemodynamics and manipulation of collaterals are equally important.

Embolism

The two most common sites of a proximal embolic source are the heart and the large arteries. Other less common sources are air, fat, cholesterol, bacteria, tumor cells, and injected drug.

Cardioembolism

The most common risk factor for cardioembolic stroke is nonvalvular atrial fibrillation. Other high-risk conditions are: sustained atrial flutter, sick sinus syndrome, left atrial and left ventricular myxoma, mitral stenosis, mechanical valve, endocarditis (infective and noninfective), recent anterior wall myocardial infarction, and dilated cardiomyopathy.

Artery-to-Artery Embolism

Emboli can originate from atherosclerotic plaques within the proximal cervicocephalic arteries or aortic arch. These emboli can cause either cerebral or retinal ischemia.

Thrombosis

Thrombotic stroke occurs as a result of obstruction of flow due to occlusive thrombus formation within the vessel wall, which is most commonly due to atherosclerotic disease. Other less common processes include dissection, vasospasm, fibromuscular dysplasia, radiation-induced vasculopathy, or moyamoya syndrome. Thrombotic occlusion can occur anywhere along the vascular bed and is generally divided into:

• Large artery atherosclerosis, or large vessel disease, involving the aorta, carotids, vertebral, and intracranial arteries.
• Small penetrating vessel thrombosis, or lacunar disease, which is strongly associated with hypertension. (Table 3.1)

Diagnosis of Stroke

As a general rule, stroke typically presents with sudden onset of focal neurologic deficits. Appropriate therapeutic interventions depend on accurately establishing the time of symptom onset, performing

Table 3.1 Incidence of Ischemic Stroke by Subtype	
Stroke Subtype	**Incidence**
Cardioembolic	30%
Atherothrombotic (large vessel) disease	30%
Lacunar (small vessel) disease	25%
Other (vasculitis, dissection, hypercoagulable state)	10%
Cryptogenic	5%

a quick and focused clinical evaluation, and rapidly evaluating brain imaging and other ancillary tests.

History

Box 3.1 Succinct Approach to the Stroke Patient

- WHERE – Neuroanatomic localization
- WHERE – Vascular localization
- WHEN – Profile of onset
- HOW – Vascular mechanism

Time of Onset

Time of symptom onset is a crucial piece of information, which will define the treatment approach. In most situations, the clinicians have to use cues, such as the time when the patient was last seen normal. The last-seen-normal time should also be used for patients who wake up with symptoms.

Evolution of Symptoms

- An abrupt onset without any preceding symptoms is highly suggestive of embolic event, whereas gradually progressive or a stuttering course with preceding stereotypical symptoms within the same vascular territory is more characteristic of thrombotic occlusion, or stenosis.
- If the patient has a fluctuating course, without returning to baseline, the time of symptom onset is considered the time of first symptom occurrence.

Accompanying Symptoms and Recent Events

- Important questions to be asked relate to the presence of headaches, which may indicate intracranial hemorrhage, dissection, or cerebral venous thrombosis.

- Other pertinent history should be tailored to identify chest pain, prior intracranial hemorrhage or strokes, head trauma, loss of consciousness, recent myocardial infarction, cardiac history, surgical history, GI bleeding, anticoagulant therapy, and co-morbid risk factors.

General Examination

Every acute stroke patient should be approached like any other acute emergency, starting with airway, breathing, and circulation assessment (ABC), vitals, and signs of trauma. If the patient does not have urgent life-threatening conditions, requiring immediate intervention, the remainder of the general exam should be focused on cardiovascular evaluation, looking for presence of arrhythmias, carotid bruits, cardiac murmurs, signs of congestive heart failure (CHF), unequal extremity pulses, and other signs that may provide important clues for stroke mechanism.

Neurological Examination

The neurological examination coupled with the history, is the most powerful diagnostic tool. The exam should focus on neuroanatomical and neurovascular localization.

A very useful and universally accepted clinical tool for assessment of acute stroke is the National Institutes of Health Stroke Scale (NIHSS) (Figure 3.2). The scale measures the level of consciousness, gaze direction, visual fields, motor and sensory functions, ataxia, language, speech, and attention. Score ranges from 0 to 42. A score above 22 signifies a severe neurological deficit, and score below 4 is consistent with a mild stroke.

- The NIHSS does not substitute the neurological examination.
- Many cranial nerve and cerebellar abnormalites can be overlooked, and thus a posterior circulation stroke can receive a relatively low score or can be totally missed. In addition, many cortical dysfunctions, such as agraphia, agraphestesia, various forms of apraxia, and agnosia are not incorporated into the scale.
- Using the scale only, without a good bedside neurological examination, can significantly minimize the severity of the clinical picture and could give a false sense of mild, or nondisabling, deficits, which could discourage aggressive treatment. Furthermore, the NIHSS should not be used as the only diagnostic tool for stroke, because other conditions may cause neurological abnormalities with high NIHSS scores.

Category	Scale definition	Score
1a. Level of Consciousness	0= Alert 1=Drowsy 2=Stuporous 3=Coma	
1b. LOC Questions (month, age)	0=Answers both correctly 1=Answer one correctly 2=Incorrect	
1c. LOC commands (open and close eyes, make a fist)	0=Obeys both correctly 1=Obeys one correctly 2=Incorrect	
2. Best gaze (patient follows examiner's finger with eyes open)	0=Normal 1=Partial gaze palsy 2=Forced deviation	
3. Visual (introduce visual stimulus in each visual field	0=Normal 1=Partial hemianopia 2=Complete hemianopia 3=Bilateral hemianopia (blind)	
4. Facial palsy (show teeth, raise eyebrows)	0=Normal 1=Minor 2=Partial 3=Complete	

Figure 3.2 The National Institutes of Health Stroke Scale (NIHSS).

5 a. Motor arm – right (Hold limb for 10 seconds)	5 b. Motor arm – left	0=No drift 1=Drift 2=Can't resist gravity 3=No effort against gravity 4=No movement UN= untestable	
		0=No drift 1=Drift 2=Can't resist gravity 3=No effort against gravity 4=No movement UN= untestable	
6 a. Motor leg – right (Hold limb for 5 seconds)	6 b. Motor leg – left	0=No drift 1=Drift 2=Can't resist gravity 3=No effort against gravity 4=No movement UN= untestable	
		0=No drift 1=Drift 2=Can't resist gravity 3=No effort against gravity 4=No movement UN= untestable	
7. Limb ataxia (finger-to-nose and heel-to-shin)		0=No ataxia 1=Present in one limb 2=Present in two limbs	
8. Sensory (light touch and pinprick in face, arm and leg)		0=Normal 1=Partial loss 2=Severe loss	

Figure 3.2 (Continued)

9. Best language (name items, describe a picture and read sentences)	0=No aphasia 1=Mild-moderate aphasia 2=Severe aphasia 3=Mute	
10. Dysarthria (evaluate speech clarity by same method as language)	0=Normal 1=Mild-moderate slurring 2=Severe (near to unitelligable) 3=Untestable	
11. Extinction and Inattention (formerly Neglect – evaluate with double simultaneous tactile and visual stimulus, ask if aware of deficits)	0=No neglect 1=Partial neglect 2=Complete neglect	
TOTAL SCORE		

The National Institutes of Health Stroke Scale (NIHSS)

Figure 3.2 (Continued)

Table 3.2 **Stroke Mimics**
Common conditions mimicking acute stroke
Hypoglycemia
Mass Lesion
Complex Migraine
Seizure with postical Todd's paralysis
Ion channels dysfunctions (channelopathies)
Psychiatric disorders with functional focal deficits

Ancillary Tests

Laboratory and Cardiac Evaluation

Recently published guidelines recommend routine tests for all patients with acute ischemic stroke, including electrolytes, glucose, complete blood count, coagulation profile, EKG, and cardiac enzymes.

- These tests can help identify stroke mimics (hypoglycemia, electrolytes disturbances) (Table 3.2) and cardiac abnormalities, such as myocardial infraction and atrial fibrillation, which are common causes of cardioembolism.

- Some laboratory abnormalities may exclude patients from thrombolytic treatment (coagulopathies), however per American Heart Association /American Stroke Association (AHA/ASA) guidelines, initiation of thrombolytic therapy should not be held if coagulation results are pending only in patients who are not on anticoagulation and do not have suspected bleeding disorder.

- Other ancillary tests such as liver function tests, urinalysis, toxicology screen, arterial blood gas, and stool guaiac are not routinely recommended and are administered on an individual basis.

  - Of note, occult GI bleeding is not an absolute contraindication for thrombolytic therapy.

Neuroimaging

Brain imaging is the only reliable diagnostic modality that can discriminate between hemorrhagic and ischemic stroke and is a mandatory test prior to initiation of any acute stroke therapy.

CT

Noncontrast head CT is the most readily available imaging modality at most hospitals. The National Institute for Neurological Disorders and Stroke (NINDS) and European Cooperative Acute Stroke Study (ECASS) III trials demonstrated that it is a useful tool for guiding intravenous thrombolysis within the first 4.5 hours after symptom onset.

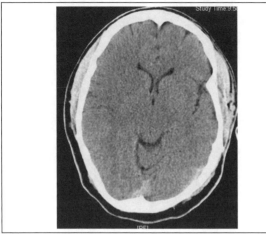

Figure 3.3 Early ischemic changes within the right insular cortex.

55

- Plain CT is very practical for detection of hemorrhage.
- CT can also detect early ischemic changes (EIC) in the hyperacute period, which can be helpful for confirming the diagnosis of ischemic stroke.
  - Presence of EIC on CT should not be used to establish time of onset or duration of ischemia, and should not discourage clinicians from administering IV thrombolysis.
  - An example of EIC is depicted in Figure 3.3. The prominent features include:
    1. Loss of grey-white matter junction, particularly in the region of the insular cortex (known as the insular ribbon sign) and the basal ganglia in cases of proximal middle cerebral artery occlusion.
    2. Effacement of the sulci in more distal territory of the affected vessel.
    These changes represent early edema and may incorporate areas of irreversible ischemia, as well as salvageable tissue.

Another important finding detected by noncontrast head CT in the hyperacute period is increased attenuation within an arterial vessel, (most commonly proximal middle cerebral artery) known as the hyperdense sign, indicative of occlusive thrombus within the vessel lumen (Figure 3.4). Vascular hyperdensities may also be noted in the basilar artery, distal internal carotid and distal middle cerebral artery (MCA) branches. However, the hyperdense sign, although highly suggestive of vascular occlusion, can be due to other factors.

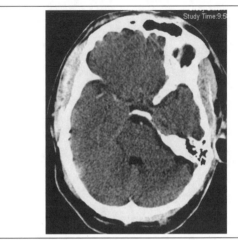

Figure 3.4 Hyperdense sign in the right middle cerebral artery, extending to the M1/M2 junction.

- The appearance of ischemic changes on CT evolves over time. After 24 hours, the ischemic zone becomes fairly hypodense and mass effect appears. Such changes on CT in a patient with reported onset within 4.5 hours should encourage the treating physicians to verify or reascertain the clinical history.

MRI

MRI is far more sensitive for ischemia than CT and equally sensitive for intraparenchymal hemorrhage. However, there are many limitations to its use in the hyperacute period.

- There are some contraindications to MRI such as, implanted devices, and poor patient cooperation or clinical instability.
- Time acquisition is longer compared with CT. With the implementation of open MRIs and abbreviated stroke protocols, some of these constraints are becoming less important.
- The diffusion-weighted sequence (DWI) can detect changes within minutes after the onset. It better delineates the location, size, and extent of the hyperacute ischemic changes (Figure 3.5).
  - Although having over 90 percent sensitivity in detection of acute ischemic stroke, DWI abnormalities can be present in other processes such as seizures, migraine, and hypoglycemia.
- Another crucial imaging finding in diagnosis of ischemia is corresponding hypointense lesion on the apparent diffusion coefficient (ADC) maps (Figure 3.6).

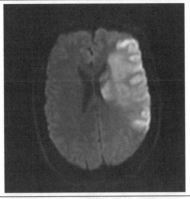

Figure 3.5 Diffusion-weighted hyperintensity (DWI) within the left middle cerebral artery territory, representing acute stroke.

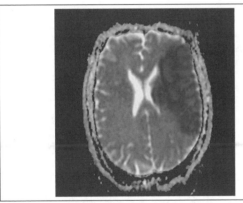

Figure 3.6 Apparent diffusion coefficient (ADC) hypointensity within the corresponding region of DWI hyperintensity in Figure 3.5

- In addition, the fluid attenuated inversion recovery (FLAIR) sequence detects the presence of old lesions, vascular hyperintensities due to slow flow, changes within the ischemic region that signify completed infarction, and provides overall excellent parenchymal visualization (Figure 3.7).
- Furthermore, conventional T1 and T2 sequences as well as gradient-recalled echo (GRE) can detect blood products as accurately as CT (Figure 3.8).

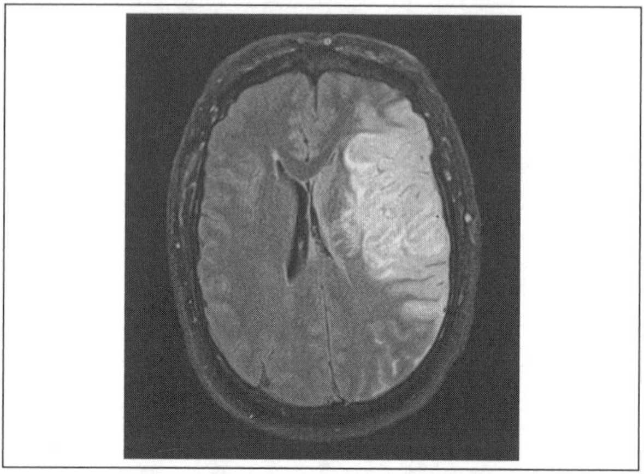

Figure 3.7 Fluid attenuated inversion recovery (FLAIR) hyperintensity within the region of DWI hyperintensity depicted in Figure 3.5, consistent with completed infarction.

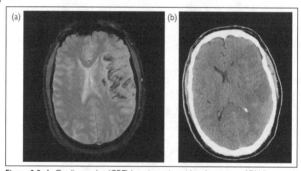

Figure 3.8 A. Gradient echo (GRE) hypointensity within the region of DWI hyperintensity depicted in Figure 3.5, consistent with hemorrhagic transformation of the ischemic infarct. B. CT scan demonstrating barely visible hemorrhagic changes in the region of DWI hyperintensity depicted in Figure 3.5, that are much better visualized on GRE.

Imaging-Based Selection for Treatment Beyond the Standard Time Windows

Multimodal Imaging

The time-based approach of the conventional intravenous (up to 4.5 hours) and intraarterial therapy (6 hours) is based on the assumption that penumbra is still present. However, the evolution of the ischemic brain tissue is highly variable from patient to patient.

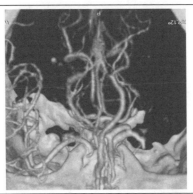

Figure 3.9 Reconstructed CTA of the intracranial circulation, demonstrating an occlusion of the left MCA stem.

- Early identification of irreversible ischemia and salvageable tissue with multimodal imaging has become the mainstay of selecting patients for acute interventions in the extended time windows.
- Visualization of the tissue and vessel status also helps to identify the stroke mechanism and etiology, which defines prognosis after intervention and can guide secondary prevention.

CTA and CT Perfusion

CTA employs a timed bolus of iodinated contrast material to make vascular structures opacify. Source images of enhanced vascular structures permit rapid identification of proximal arterial occlusion (Figure 3.9).

CTP utilizes iodinated material to track the passage of contrast-labeled blood through the brain. Acquisition of serial images permits the generation of time-intensity curves for contrast passage through the brain. Perfusion maps are then constructed and various hemo-dynamic perfusion parameters including mean transit time (MTT) cerebral blood volume (CBV), and cerebral blood flow (CBF) are delineated (Figure 3.10).

- CTP lesions with CBV values under 2.3 ml/100 g or 65 percent are generally considered equivalent to diffusion-weighted imaging (DWI) lesions in representing irreversible ischemia.
- The ischemic penumbra on CTP is defined as a mismatch between a CBV < 2.3 ml/100 g, and a relative mean transit time (MTT) prolongation > 145 percent.
- CTA/CTP imaging paradigm has the advantage of quick acquisition time and widespread availability. However, CTP can only be acquired in the specific region of interest as

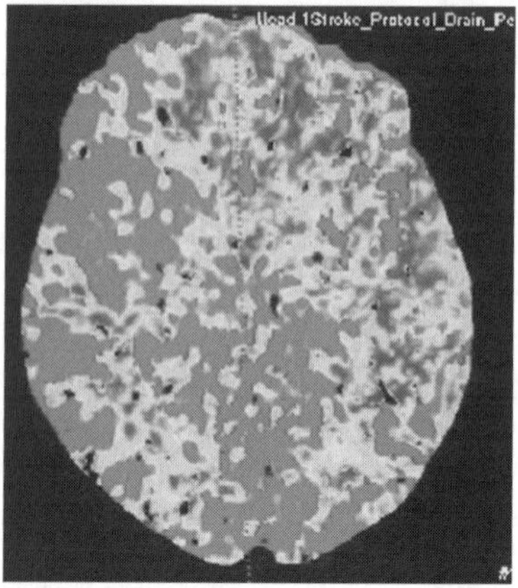

Figure 3.10 Perfusion-weighted CT, demonstrating decreased blood flow within the anterior portion of the left MCA and bilateral ACA territories.

opposed to perfusion-weighted image (PWI) parameters, which can be visualized over larger areas. The other disadvantage of multimodal CT is its inability to detect the presence of microbleeds, lacunar disease, and ischemic changes in the posterior fossa; and the need to use iodinated contrast.

MRA and MR perfusion

In addition to the advantages of MRI in detection of acute ischemia, magnetic resonance angiography (MRA) and PWI may provide additional information regarding vessel status, collateral flow, and territories at risk. PWI typically employs gadolinium and the dynamic acquisition of serial images to track the influx of contrast-labeled blood into the brain to define areas of hypoperfusion. The diffusion-perfusion mismatch has been widely used as a conceptual model to capture or identify the ischemic penumbra (Figures 3.11, 3.12, and 3.13).

Figure 3.14 provides an algorithm for suggested management of patients with acute stroke.

Therapeutic Strategies in Acute Ischemic Stroke

Recanalization

- Recanalization is the single most powerful treatment in acute ischemic stroke (Molina and Saver, 2005). Figure 3.15 provides an algorithm for recanalization strategies.

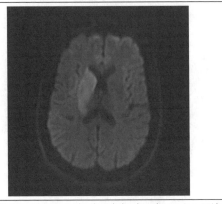

Figure 3.11 DWI hyperintensity within the right basal ganglia, consistent with acute infarct.

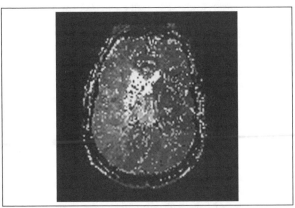

Figure 3.12 Perfusion-weighted images (PWI), demonstrating hypoperfusion of the entire right MCA territory, much larger than the DWI lesion depicted in Figure 3.11. The difference between the PWI and DWI volumes represents an area of reversible ischemia.

Intravenous Thrombolytic Therapy

Intravenous recombinant tissue plasminogen activator (tPA) is the standard of care in the United States for patients with acute stroke within three hours of symptom onset. This limited time window was based on the NINDS tPA Stroke Study.

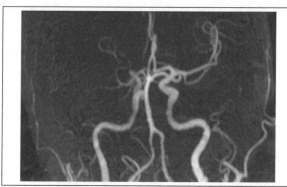

Figure 3.13 MRA of the intracranial vessels, demonstrating a right MCA occlusion with a corresponding zones of distal hypoperfusion and ischemic stroke, depicted in Figures 3.11 and 3.12.

In that study, 39 percent of tPA-treated patients and 26 percent of the placebo group achieved functional independence. This translated to a number needed to treat of 8 for 1 additional patient to achieve minimal or no disability. The number of patients who suffered the most feared complication of symptomatic intracranial hemorrhage (sICH) was 6.6 percent. However, detailed analysis of the trial, suggested that the number needed to treat to contribute to *any* improvement may be as low as 3. Thus, for every 100 patients treated with IV tPA, 32 benefit, and only 3 may be harmed.

Recently, the results of the European Acute Stroke Study (ECASS) III demonstrated that intravenous thrombolysis administered within 4.5 hours of symptoms onset is still safe and beneficial. The exclusion criteria were similar to the NINDS study, with 4 additional exlusions:

1. Age > 80 years
2. No combination of prior stroke plus diabetes
3. Severe stroke (NIHSS > 25 or > 1/3 of MCA territory by imaging
4. Any concurrent use of warfarin (regardless of the INR)

The results of ECASS III led to a release of an official recommendation from the stroke council of AHA/ASA, encouraging physicians to offer IV TPA to patients with strokes within 4.5 hours who meet ECASS III inclusion/exclusion criteria.

Rapid administration of IV rt-TPA is the key for successful treatment. The likelihood of favorable outcome diminishes as the time to initiation of thrombolysis increases. A guide for minimizing the door-to-needle time for emergent evaluation of acute stroke was established by NINDS in 1997 (Table 3.3).

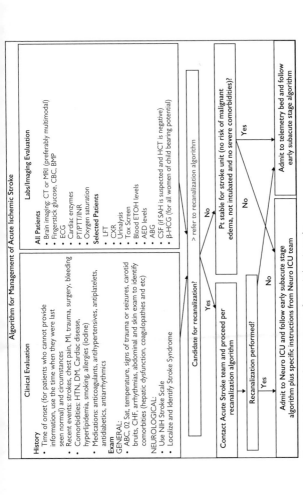

Figure 3.14 Algorithm for management of acute ischemic stroke

Algorithm for Recanalization in Acute Ischemic Stroke

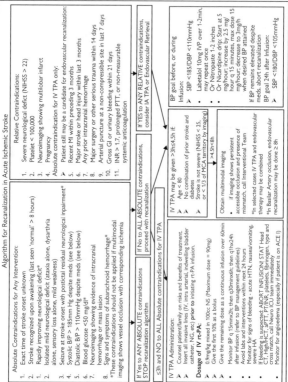

Absolute Contraindications for Any Intervention:
1. Exact time of stroke onset unknown
2. Stroke recognized upon awakening (last seen 'normal' > 8 hours)
1. Rapidly improving neurological deficit*
2. Isolated mild neurological deficit (ataxia alone, dysarthria alone, sensory loss alone, mild weakness)
3. Seizure at stroke onset with postictal residual neurological impairment*
4. Systolic B/P > 185mm Hg despite meds (see below)
5. Diastolic B/P > 110mmHg despite meds (see below)
6. Blood glucose <50 mg/dl*
7. Neuroimaging showing evidence of intracranial hemorrhage or mass lesion
8. Signs and symptoms of subarachnoid hemorrhage*
*These contraindications should not be applied if multimodal imaging shows vessel occlusion with corresponding ischemia

Relative Contraindications:
1. Severe neurological deficit (NIHSS > 22)
2. Platelet < 100,000
3. Neuroimaging showing multilobar infarct
4. Pregnancy
Absolute contraindication for IV TPA only:
5. Recent MI within preceding 3 months
6. Major stroke or head injury within last 3 months
7. Any prior intracranial hemorrhage
8. Major surgery or other serious trauma within 14 days
9. Arterial puncture at a non-compressible site in last 7 days
10. Gross GI or urinary bleeding within 21 days
11. INR > 1.7, prolonged PTT, or non-measurable systemic anticoagulation

Absolute contraindication for endovascular recanalization:
➤ Patient still may be a candidate for endovascular recanalization:

If YES to ANY RELATIVE contraindications, consider IA TPA or Endovascular Retrieval

If Yes to ANY ABSOLUTE contraindications, STOP recanalization algorithm

If No to ALL ABSOLUTE contraindications, proceed with recanalization

≤3h and NO to ALL Absolute contraindications for IV TPA

IV TPA may be given >3hs4.5h if:
➤ Age < 80
➤ No combination of prior stroke and diabetes
➤ Stroke is not severe (NIHSS < 25, or < 1/3 of MCA territory by imaging)

>4.5h-8h

Obtain multimodal imaging
* if imaging shows persistent accessible occlusion and presence of mismatch, call Interventional Team
*In selected cases IV TPA and endovascular therapy may be combined
*In Basilar Artery occlusion, endovascular recanalization may be done ≥ 8h

IV TPA Administration:
➤ Counsel patient/family on risks and benefits of treatment.
➤ Insert all invasive lines (IV, intra arterial, indwelling bladder catheter, NG, etc) **prior to initiating rt-PA infusion.**
Dosage of IV rt-PA:
➤ 0.9mg/kg in 100cc NS (Maximum dose = 90mg)
➤ Give the first 10% as a bolus
➤ Give the remaining dose as a continuous infusion over 60min
• Monitor BP q 15min x2h; then q30min x6h; then q1h x24h after infusion (refer to BP management guidelines)
• Avoid labs and interventions within next 24 hours
• Monitor for signs of bleeding - acute HTN, nausea/vomiting, severe HA
• If bleeding is suspected: ABORT INFUSION! STAT Head CT, Hgb/HCT, aPTT, PT/INR, platelets, fibrinogen, type and cross match. Call Neuro ICU team immediately
• Monitor for angioedema (especially if patient is on ACE I)

BP goal before, or during Infusion:
➤ SBP <185/DBP <110mmHg
• Labetalol 10mg IVP over 1-2min, may repeat once
• Or Nitropaste 1-2 inches
• Or Nicardipine drip: Start at 5 mg/hour; increase by 2.5 mg/hour q 15 minutes, max dose 15 mg/hour; decrease to 3mg/h when desired BP attained
If BP remains elevated despite meds abort infusion
BP goal 24h after Infusion:
➤ SBP <180/DBP <105mmHg

Figure 3.14 Algorithm for Recanalization in Acute Ischemic Stroke

Table 3.3 **Recommended Target time points for evaluation of acute stroke patients.**

Time from ED arrival	Action
10 minutes	Evaluate potential stroke patient (ED physician)
15 minutes	Notify stroke team or physician with stroke expertise
25 minutes	Initiate head CT
45 minutes	Interpret head CT
60 minutes	Administer IV tPA

Adapted with permission from The National Institute of Neurological Disorders and Stroke (NINDS) rt-PA Stroke Study Group. Stroke 1997; 28: 1530–1540.

If the patient is deemed eligible for treatment, the tPA should be administered as follows:

- 0.9 mg/kg mixed in 100 cc normal saline (NS) (Maximum dose = 90 mg)
- Give the first 10 percent as a bolus.
- Give the remaining dose as a continuous infusion over 60 minutes.

There are some important points about the selection criteria for acute thrombolysis:

- Head CT is necessary for exclusion of intracranial hemorrhage. However, when the clinical diagnosis is unclear, additional imaging, such as MRI with DWI or CT/CTA/CT perfusion may be helpful.
- NIHSS does not represent the true neurological exam, and low score for disabling deficits, such as aphasia alone or hemianopia alone should not discourage treatment.
- Hyperglycemia has been associated with increased risk of hemorrhage and poor outcome. Therefore, patients with elevated serum glucose > 400 mg/dl may need to be approached on a case-by-case basis.
- Presence of myocardial infarction may be safe, as long as cleared by cardiology. However, if signs and symptoms of pericarditis are present, there is a risk of hemopericardium.
- Seizure at the onset may not be a contraindication if CTA or MRI can confirm stroke, as the neurological deficits may not be due to postictal Todd's paralysis.
- Early ischemic changes on CT should not be considered as a contraindication for treatment. Only presence of frank hypodensity, involving a large or extensive area, should be considered contraindicative.

- Consent is not required because IV tPA is considered a standard of care up to **3 hours from onset**. However, discussion with the patient and family members should take place.
- Blood pressures may be lowered only by nonaggressive measures. The AHA/ASA guidelines for blood pressure management before and during infusion are listed below:
  - BP goal before, or during infusion: SBP <185/DBP <110 mmHg
  - BP goal 24 hours after infusion: SBP <180/DBP <105 mmHg

Patient monitoring and management during and after treatment should include the following:

- Monitor BP q15min × 2 hours; then q30min × 6 hours; then q1hours × 24 hours after infusion.
- Avoid labs and interventions within next 24 hours.
- Monitor for signs of bleeding, acute hypertension nausea/vomiting, severe headache.
- Monitor for angioedema (especially if patient is on angiotensin converting enzyme – inhibitors, ACE-I).

Management of complication during and after infusion should include the following:

- Management of symptomatic intracranial hemorrhage associated with IV tPA use:
  - Any worsening of clinical or neurological status, new neurological deficits, acute hypertension, nausea, vomiting, new-onset headaches, as well as new-onset seizures should alert the clinician about potential hemorrhage.
  - Treatment recommendation by AHA/ASA are mainly based on NINDS trial protocol and outlined in Figure 3.16.
- Management of angioedema associated with IV-TPA
  - Incidence: 1-2 percent in patients treated with IV-TPA.
  - It is more common in patients taking ACE-I.
  - Usually starts near the end of infusion.
    1. Begin examining the tongue 20 minute before the end of infusion. Look for tongue swelling.
    2. If angioedema is suspected, immediately:
       a. Consider early discontinuation of rt-TPA infusion.
       b. Administer diphenhydramine 50 mg IV.
       c. Administer ranitidine 50 mg IV or famotidine 20 mg IV.
    3. If tongue continues to enlarge:
       a. Give methylprednisolone 80 mg to 100 mg IV.
    4. If there is any further increase of angioedema:
       a. Administer epinephrine 0.1 percent 0.3 m SQ or by nebulizer 0.5 ml.

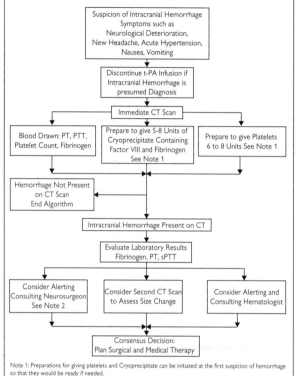

The following algorithm was developed for using during a clinical trial. All or part of this algorithm may be adapted for use of thrombolytic therapy of stroke for approved indications. The application of this algorithm may have to be modified in order to function with resources available in a particular location.

Suspicion of Intracranial Hemorrhage
Symptoms such as
Neurological Deterioration,
New Headache, Acute Hypertension,
Nausea, Vomiting

Discontinue t-PA Infusion if
Intracranial Hemorrhage is
presumed Diagnosis

Immediate CT Scan

Blood Drawn: PT, PTT, Platelet Count, Fibrinogen

Prepare to give 5-8 Units of Cryoprecipitate Containing Factor VIII and Fibrinogen See Note 1

Prepare to give Platelets 6 to 8 Units See Note 1

Hemorrhage Not Present on CT Scan
End Algorithm

Intracranial Hemorrhage Present on CT

Evaluate Laboratory Results
Fibrinogen, PT, sPTT

Consider Alerting Consulting Neurosurgeon See Note 2

Consider Second CT Scan to Assess Size Change

Consider Alerting and Consulting Hematologist

Consensus Decision:
Plan Surgical and Medical Therapy

Note 1: Preparations for giving platelets and Cryoprecipitate can be initiated at the first suspicion of hemorrhage so that they would be ready if needed.
Note 2: It is highly recommended to have a plan for obtaining neurosurgical advice.

Figure 3.16 Management of symptomatic intracranial hemorrhage associated with IV tPA use. Reprinted with permission from the UCLA Stroke Center.

b. Call Anesthesiology/ENT or any appropriate in-house services STAT for possible emergency cricotomy/ tracheostomy or fiberoptic nasotracheal intubation if oral intubation is unsuccessful.

Tongue large but oral intubation possible

Tongue too large for orotracheal intubation

Severe stridor impending airway obstruction

Perform orotracheal intubation STAT

Perform fiberoptic nasotracheal intubation

Perform tracheostomy

Endovascular Recanalization Strategies

Intra-arterial Thrombolysis

Large clots, leading to proximal arterial occlusions, as in the terminal internal carotid artery, or proximal middle cerebral artery, may not recanalize with systemic thrombolysis. In these cases, locally administered intra-arterial thrombolysis may offer additional advantages.

- The Prolyse in Acute Cerebral Thromboembolism II trial (PROACT II) was the only randomized clinical trial that demonstrated substantial clinical benefit of intra-arterial thrombolysis alone, initiated within six hours of onset of a proximal MCA (M1 or M2) occlusion.
- Patients with history of recent surgery or interventional procedures, GI bleeding, head trauma, intracranial hemorrhage, mild coagulopathy, as well as pregnant women in whom intravenous thrombolysis is contraindicated may be candidates for intra-arterial therapy.

Mechanical Revascularization

Multiple novel endovascular catheter-based approaches for mechanical recanalization have emerged in the past decade. The devices used can be divided in two major categories: (1) thrombectomy via clot retrieval or suction aspiration; (2) mechanical lysis and reperfusion via angioplasty/stenting.

- Mechanical revascularization can be used alone or in combination with intra-arterial thrombolysis for the indications listed earlier.

Combined Intravenous and Intra-arterial Therapy

The combination of intravenous and intraarterial approach offers the advantage of rapid initiation of systemic thrombolysis, with subsequent local administration of thrombolytic drug or mechanical manipulation, which, theoretically, would lead to higher recanalization rates.

Basilar Artery Occlusion

Basilar artery occlusion represents a unique entity in acute ischemic stroke due to the very high mortality rates and extremely poor functional outcome in the event of survival.

- All patients with sudden onset of unexplained stupor or coma and/or preceding signs and symptoms of vertebrobasilar ischemia should be evaluated with rapid imaging of the posterior circulation (MRA or CTA).
  - The time window for recanalization in such cases is not clearly defined. However, multiple small series and case reports indicated relatively good outcome of basilar artery recanalization, beyond the standard time windows for intravenous or intraarterial thrombolysis.

- These patients should be treated aggressively either with IV tPA within 4.5 hours of onset, or with endovascular therapies, such as mechanical thrombectomy or intraarterial clot lysis up to 12 hours from onset.

Angioplasty and Stenting

Intracranial angioplasty and stenting is a promising endovascular treatment, particularly in patients with occlusion or critical stenosis due to atherosclerotic disease with superimposed in situ thrombosis. Carotid stenting of cervical carotid occlusion can also be performed acutely in the setting of acute stroke.

Collateral flow augmentation

Dedicated approaches to augment collateral flow are currently being developed. Anecdotal reports suggest that hypervolemic and/ or hypertensive therapy for flow augmentation and reperfusion in patients with acute ischemic stroke may be beneficial in patients with large vessel occlusive disease and fluctuating neurologic deficits. The length of time and the optimal target blood pressure is not defined. Similarly, the decision to proceed with hypervolemic versus hypertensive therapy depends on individual patient factors. Overall, optimal hydration is required.

Another novel and promising strategy is catheter-based collateral flow augmentation, applied in the acute period. An intra-aortic balloon known as the NeuroFlo™ has been demonstrated to augment cerebral perfusion, and is currently undergoing further safety and potential efficacy studies.

Neuroprotection

Neuroprotective strategies have been mainly focused on blockage of the apoptotic cascade and prolongation of neuronal survival. However, over the past several decades multiple clinical trials of neuroprotection in acute ischemic strokes have failed. Ultra-early treatment initiated in the ambulance en route may buy time for reperfusion. A clinical trial, the Field Administration of Stroke Therapy-Magnesium (FAST-MAG) trial, based at UCLA, utilizes IV magnesium sulfate administered in the field as a potential therapy.

Transient Ischemic Attack

Since the introduction of MRI with DWI and PWI sequences, the definition of transient ischemic attack (TIA) has evolved. The classic time-based definition was "any focal cerebral or retinal ischemic event with symptoms lasting less than 24 hours." Recently, however, multiple studies have demonstrated that up to 50 percent of patients with classically defined TIA show brain injury on MRI. Thus, using pathophysiologic, rather than time criterion, AHA/ASA endorsed a new, tissue-based definition of TIA:

Transient Episode of Neurological Dysfunction, Caused by Focal Brain, Spinal Cord, or Retinal Ischemia, without Acute Infarction

- AHA/ASA recommends the term *acute neurovascular syndrome* for patients with relatively minor symptoms of short duration who do not receive a detailed diagnostic evaluation.
- The diagnosis of TIA should be considered only if the transient neurologic event is potentially referable to a specific cerebrovascular territory.
- Proper clinical judgment should be used prior to ordering costly work-up because not every transient neurologic deficit falls under the spectrum of the neurovascular syndromes.

The principal pathophysiologic mechanism of TIA is the same as ischemic stroke.

- Transient deficits referable to different arterial territories are highly suggestive of cardiac source.
- Stereotypical episodes within the same vascular territory can be due to either emboli from an ulcerated plaque or from flow-limiting stenosis, or a combination of both.
- Important clues that could help identify the mechanism are clinical correlation with hemodynamic variables, such as blood pressure, orthosasis (limb-shaking TIA), and intravascular volume changes.

TIA: the Warning of Stroke

It has long been recognized that TIA can portend stroke. The risk of stroke is particularly high in the short-term, with most studies indicating more than 10 percent risk in 90 days and up to 4 percent within the first 24 hours,. Risk of major cardiac events is also elevated in patients experiencing TIA and accounts for 2.6 percent of hospital-ization rates within 90 days.

Risk Stratification

The most validated method of stratifying stroke risk after TIA is the ABCD2 scoring system (Table 3.4).

Diagnostic Evaluation

- **The diagnostic approach to TIA is similar to the evaluation of ischemic stroke.**
- The utility of noncontrast head CT in evaluation of TIA has little value in identification of ischemia within the hyperacute period.

Table 3.4 ABCD² Score for Stroke Risk Assessment After TIA.

ABCD2 Score for TIA	
Age ≥ 60?	1
BP ≥ 140/90 mmHg at initial evaluation	1
Clinical features: Unilateral weakness	2
Clinical features: Speech disturbance without weakness	1
Diabetes Mellitus	1
Duration of Symptoms 10–59 minutes	1
Duration of Symptoms > 60 minutes	2

Notes:

• 0–3 points: Low Risk

• 2-day stroke risk: 1.0%

• 7-day stroke risk: 1.2%

• 90-day stroke risk: 3.1%

It is reasonable to hospitalize patients if score is:

• ≥3

• 0–2 and diagnostic work up cannot be completed within 48 hours

• 0–2 and other evidence of cerebral ischemia

Source: Reprinted with permission from Rothwell et al., 2005; Johnston et al., 2007; Josephson et al., 2008.

- Conventional MRI is far more sensitive than standard CT in identifying new and pre-existing ischemic lesions. Numerous studies have demonstrated that identification of DWI positivity with frequency ranging from 25 percent to 67% percent is of substantial clinical utility in patients with TIAs.

- Patients with TIAs should have a detailed evaluation of the intracranial and extracranial circulation.

- Cardioembolic source has been reported in 6 –10 percent of patients presenting with TIAs.

- All patients should have ECG as soon as possible after TIA.

- Inpatient telemetry or Holter monitoring is useful in detection of paroxysmal atrial fibrillation in patients with highly suspected embolic source of unclear origin.

- Transthoracic echocardiography (TTE) is reasonable in evaluation of patients with TIAs. However, transesophageal echocardiography (TEE) is more sensitive for detection of proximal embolic source, aortic arch atheroma, atrial septal abnormalities, atrial thrombi, and valvular disease.

Suggested Readings

Astrup J, Siesjo, BK, et al. Thresholds in cerebral ischemia—the ischemic penumbra. *Stroke* 1981;12(6):723–725.

Babikian VL, Caplan LR. Brain embolism is a dynamic process with variable characteristics. *Neurology.* 2000;54(4):797–801.

Baird AE, Warach S. Magnetic resonance imaging of acute stroke. *J Cereb Blood Flow Metab.* 1998;18(6):583–609.

Bhardwaj A, Alkayed NJ, et al. Mechanisms of ischemic brain damage. *Curr Cardiol. Rep.* 2003;5(2):160–167.

Bogousslavsky J, Hachinski, VC, et al. Clinical predictors of cardiac and arterial lesions in carotid transient ischemic attacks. *Arch Neurol.* 1986;43(3):229–233.

Bogousslavsky J, Hachinski, VC, et al. Cardiac and arterial lesions in carotid transient ischemic attacks. *Arch Neurol.* 1986;43(3):223–228.

Bose A, Henkes H, et al. The Penumbra System: a mechanical device for the treatment of acute stroke due to thromboembolism. *AJNR Am J Neuroradiol.* 2008;29(7):1409–1413.

Easton JD, Saver JL, et al. Definition and evaluation of transient ischemic attack: a scientific statement for healthcare professionals from the American Heart Association/American Stroke Association Stroke Council; Council on Cardiovascular Surgery and Anesthesia; Council on Cardiovascular Radiology and Intervention; Council on Cardiovascular Nursing; and the Interdisciplinary Council on Peripheral Vascular Disease. The American Academy of Neurology affirms the value of this statement as an educational tool for neurologists. *Stroke.* 2009;40(6):2276–2293.

Elkins JS, Sidney S, et al. Electrocardiographic findings predict short-term cardiac morbidity after transient ischemic attack. *Arch Neurol.* 2002;59(9):1437–1441.

Furlan A, Higashida R, et al. Intra-arterial prourokinase for acute ischemic stroke. The PROACT II study: a randomized controlled trial. Prolyse in Acute Cerebral Thromboembolism. *JAMA.* 1999;282(21):2003–2011.

Hacke W, Kaste W, et al. Thrombolysis with alteplase 3 to 4.5 hours after acute ischemic stroke. *N Engl J Med.* 2008;359(13):1317–1329.

Hankey GJ, Slattery JM, et al. The prognosis of hospital-referred transient ischaemic attacks. *J Neurol Neurosurg Psychiatry.* 1991;54(9):793–802.

Johnston SC, Rothwell PM, et al. Validation and refinement of scores to predict very early stroke risk after transient ischaemic attack. *Lancet.* 2007;369(9558):283–292.

Josephson SA, Sidney S, et al. Higher ABCD2 score predicts patients most likely to have true transient ischemic attack. *Stroke.* 2008;39(11):3096–3098.

Kernan WN, Feinstein AR, et al. A methodological appraisal of research on prognosis after transient ischemic attacks. *Stroke.* 1991;22(9):1108–1116.

Kidwell CS, Chalela JA, et al. Comparison of MRI and CT for detection of acute intracerebral hemorrhage. *JAMA.* 2004;292(15):1823–1830.

Levy EI, Siddiqui AH, et al. First Food and Drug Administration-approved prospective trial of primary intracranial stenting for acute stroke:

SARIS (stent-assisted recanalization in acute ischemic stroke). *Stroke.* 2009;40(11):3552–3556.

Liebeskind DS. Understanding blood flow: the other side of an acute arterial occlusion. *Int J Stroke.* 2007;2(2):118–120.

Molina CA, Saver JL. Extending reperfusion therapy for acute ischemic stroke: emerging pharmacological, mechanical, and imaging strategies. *Stroke.* 2005;36(10):2311–2320.

Nedeltchev K, Remonda, L, et al. (2004). Acute stenting and thromboaspiration in basilar artery occlusions due to embolism from the dominating vertebral artery. *Neuroradiology.* 2004;46(8):686–691.

Rordorf G, Koroshetz WJ, et al. A pilot study of drug-induced hypertension for treatment of acute stroke. *Neurology.* 2001;56(9):1210–1213.

Rordorf G, Cramer SC, et al. (1997). Pharmacological elevation of blood pressure in acute stroke. Clinical effects and safety. *Stroke.* 1997;28(11):2133–2138.

Rothwell PM, Giles, MF, et al. A simple score (ABCD) to identify individuals at high early risk of stroke after transient ischaemic attack. *Lancet.* 2005;366(9479):2936.

Saver JL. Number needed to treat estimates incorporating effects over the entire range of clinical outcomes: novel derivation method and application to thrombolytic therapy for acute stroke. *Arch Neurol.* 2004;61(7):1066–1070.

Saver JL, Kidwell C, et al. Prehospital neuroprotective therapy for acute stroke: results of the Field Administration of Stroke Therapy-Magnesium (FAST-MAG) pilot trial. *Stroke.* 2004;35(5):e106–e108.

Schlaug G, Benfield A, et al. The ischemic penumbra: operationally defined by diffusion and perfusion MRI. *Neurology.* 1999;53(7):1528–1537.

Smith WS, Sung G, et al. Mechanical thrombectomy for acute ischemic stroke: final results of the Multi MERCI trial. *Stroke.* 2008;39(4):1205–1212.

Strandberg M, Marttila RJ, et al. (2002). Transoesophageal echocardiography in selecting patients for anticoagulation after ischaemic stroke or transient ischaemic attack. *J Neurol Neurosurg Psychiatry.* 2002;73(1):29–33.

The National Institute of Neurological Disorders and Stroke (NINDS) rt-PA Stroke Study Group. A Systems Approach to Immediate Evaluation and Management of Hyperacute Stroke Experience at Eight Centers and Implications for Community Practice and Patient Care. *Stroke.* 1997;28:1530–1540.

Tissue plasminogen activator for acute ischemic stroke. The National Institute of Neurological Disorders and Stroke rt-PA Stroke Study Group. *N Engl J Med.* 1995;333(24):1581–1587.

Wintermark M, Flanders AE, et al. Perfusion-CT assessment of infarct core and penumbra: receiver operating characteristic curve analysis in 130 patients suspected of acute hemispheric stroke. *Stroke.* 2006;37(4):979–985.

Chapter 4

Cerebral Hemorrhage

Joshua N. Goldstein and Jonathan Rosand

Intracerebral Hemorrhage

Intracerebral hemorrhage (ICH) accounts for approximately 15 percent of strokes, but carries the highest morbidity and mortality of any stroke subtype. ICH can be primary or secondary.

Causes

- Primary ICH most commonly occurs in individuals >55 years.
  - Primary ICH typically results from the rupture of a small caliber cerebral artery or arteriole that has been affected by a chronic vasculopathy, such as cerebral amyloid angiopathy or so-called hypertensive vasculopathy.
  - Deep location (thalamus, basal ganglia) is most often attributed to effects of chronic hypertension (Figure 4.1). Other common sites of hypertensive hemorrhage are the pons and cerebellum.
  - Lobar (cortical-subcortical) location is most often attributed to effects of cerebral amyloid angiopathy (Figure 4.2). Note, however, that there can be overlap.
- Secondary ICH:
  - Ruptured aneurysm
  - Arteriovenous malformation (AVM)
  - Tumor
  - Cerebral venous sinus thrombosis (CVST)
  - Moyamoya disease (and other vascular abnormalities)
  - Drug intoxication (e.g., acute cocaine use) can also cause ICH
  - Trauma
  - Coagulopathy

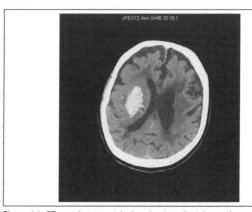

Figure 4.1 CT scan showing a right deep basal ganglionic hemorrhage.

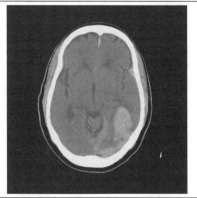

Figure 4.2 CT scan showing a left lobar parieto-occipital hemorrhage likely due to amyloid angiopathy.

This chapter will discuss the various types of ICH in distinct sections.

History

- Abrupt onset of severe headache
- Vomiting
- Any focal or generalized neurological symptom
- Seizure

Important factors to obtain in the history include:

- Age of patient
- Time of onset, or time last seen normal (patients presenting early are at higher risk for early hematoma expansion)
- Rapidity of onset of headache
- Co-existent symptoms at onset (diplopia, syncope, weakness, or other neurological symptoms)
- Seizure at onset
- Past medical history, including hypertension and premorbid neurologic and cognitive status
- Family history, including aneurysms or AV malformations
- Medications, including anticoagulants, antiplatelets, and antiepileptics
- Social history, including history of alcohol abuse and drugs of abuse (such as cocaine)

Physical Examination

- Any new onset focal or generalized neurological deficit.
- Neurological examination can be normal, especially in subarachnoid hemorrhage (SAH). Patients with SAH may only exhibit:

- Third nerve palsy.
- Meningismus.
- Subhyaloid hemorrhage on funduscopic examination.

Important factors to examine include:

- Airway, breathing, and pulse.
- External signs of head trauma.
- Focused neurologic examination including Glasgow Coma Scale Score. It is important to document this so that the patient can be followed for early signs of neurological deterioration.

Work-up

- Emergency cranial imaging is essential in all patients with suspected ICH. Noncontrast CT is almost always the initial study performed.
- Brain MRI, with or without gadolinium, and cerebrovascular imaging, including CT angiography, catheter angiography, or CT or MR venography may be necessary (depending on the details of the case) for differentiating primary vs. secondary ICH.
  - Patients with lobar ICH, intraventricular blood, and younger age have higher rates of underlying vascular malformation.
  - ICH immediately adjacent to the subarachnoid space at the base of the brain or basal interhemispheric fissure can be due to a ruptured saccular aneurysm.
  - Hemorrhage secondary to ischemic stroke may show signs of surrounding cytotoxic edema conforming to an arterial territory.
  - Hemorrhage associated with tumor may appear complex, with a heterogeneous appearance, or more surrounding vasogenic edema than might be expected with primary ICH.
  - Multifocal hemorrhages, especially in nonarterial distributions, are worrisome for underlying venous sinus thrombosis.
- CT angiography (CTA) produces high quality images of the larger arterial vessels, and is often rapidly available in the emergency setting.
- MRI/MRA is particularly valuable if underlying tumor or other etiology is suspected. MRA can also evaluate the vasculature.
- Digital subtraction angiography (DSA) is, in some centers, considered the definitive test to rule out an underlying vascular abnormality.
- CT venography (CTV) or MR venography (MRV) should be considered if CVST is under consideration.

Primary ICH Management

Airway

Emergency airway management requires balancing the risk of losing the patient's airway vs. losing the ability to perform the neurologic exam. For those patients requiring endotracheal intubation, those in the emergency setting are typically candidates for rapid sequence intubation, whereas those who have been in the hospital for some time undergoing urgent rather than emergent intubation may be candidates for use of induction agents (such as etomidate, propofol, or midazolam). In this situation, document the pre-intubation neurological exam.

- Rapid Sequence Intubation:
  - Pretreatment medications: Consider Lidocaine 1.5 mg/kg (may blunt a rise in ICP associated with intubation).
  - Induction: Consider Etomidate (may preserve cerebral perfusion pressure [CPP]) 0.3 mg/kg.
  - Paralysis: Consider Succinylcholine (1.5 mg/kg), Rocuronium (1 mg/kg), or Vecuronium (0.15 mg/kg).

Sedation

Consider propofol (5–80 mcg/kg/min) as a continuous drip for sedation. The goal is to provide effective sedation while retaining the ability to follow a neurologic exam in the acute phase.

Ventilation

Mechanical ventilation should minimize positive end-expiratory pressure (PEEP) and high peak inspiratory pressure (PIP) to avoid increasing venous congestion in the brain. Typical initial settings are 100 percent FiO_2, a ventilatory rate of 10–12 breaths per minute, and a tidal volume of approximately 10 cc/kg. Hyperventilation can reduce ICP in the short term only and should be reserved for patients with impending or active herniation who require operative management.

Prevention of Hematoma Expansion

Among patients with primary ICH, as many as 40 percent experience ongoing bleeding in hospital, resulting in hematoma expansion. The initial 24 hours after symptom onset is the highest risk period. Therapies aimed at reducing this risk may improve outcomes (though this has not been proven):

- Blood pressure (BP) management.
  - One clinical trial showed that reducing SBP<140 in the acute phase reduced the risk of hematoma expansion (although no difference in neurologic outcome was found).

- AHA recommendations:
  - If there is suspicion for elevated ICP and either SBP>180 or mean arterial pressure (MAP) >130, reduce SBP below 180 but maintain CPP>60–80 mmHg.
  - If there is no suspicion of elevated ICP, then the goal should be for SBP<160.
- European Stroke Initiative recommendations:
  - If there is a history of hypertension, and BP>180/105, then consider lowering below 170/100.
  - If there is no history of hypertension, and BP>160/95, then consider lowering below 150/90.
  - Do not lower MAP by more than 20 percent in the acute phase.
- BP agents of choice:
  - Labetalol: Intermittent boluses of 10–40 mg, or continuous drop (2–8 mg/min).
  - Esmolol: 500 mcg/kg load, then 50–200 mcg/kg/min maintenance.
  - Nicardipine: 5–15 mg/hour.
  - Hydralazine: 10–20 mg q4–6 hours.
  - Nitroprusside: 0.5–10 mcg/kg/min.
  - Enalapril: 0.625–1.2 mg q6 hours.
  - Nitroprusside is being used less frequently because it can increase ICP and because there are other, newer agents that have a better side effect profile.
- Hemostatic therapy
  - Although some centers use activated Factor VIIa off-label to reduce the risk of hematoma expansion, this therapy has not been shown to improve neurologic outcome.
- Anticoagulation reversal
  - Patients on oral anticoagulants are at higher risk of hematoma expansion, and this expansion can be more delayed. Acute anticoagulation reversal is recommended.
  - **Warfarin**:
    - Deliver IV vitamin K, 5–10 mg (avoid subcutaneous or intramuscular forms, which are minimally effective).
    - Provide factor repletion, which may improve hemostasis in the acute phase while awaiting an effect of vitamin K:
      - Prothrombin complex concentrate (PCC), depending on the agent, can provide most or all the missing factors, and reverse the international normalized ratio (INR) in minutes. Dosing depends on the agent; contact your blood bank for which agent is available at your hospital.

- Activated Factor VIIa (NovoSeven): Reverses the INR in minutes. There is no consistently agreed upon dose; some centers use 40 mcg/kg as a one-time intravenous dose.
- Fresh Frozen Plasma (FFP): Requires hours to obtain and deliver, but it is widely available in most hospitals. Dosing can start at 15 ml/kg—note that up to 2L may be required in practice.
- Check the INR immediately after factor repletion, then every 6 hours for 24 hours. When using activated Factor VII or a PCC, it is important to follow this up with FFP.
- **Heparin**:
  - Consider protamine 10–50 mg IV.
- **Platelet disorders**:
  - Thrombocytopenia (platelet count < 100,000/μL): Consider platelet transfusion.
  - Von Willebrand syndromes: Administer 0.3 mcg/kg DDAVP IV over 30 minutes, and consider VWF factor concentrate.
  - Some centers advocate the use of 1 dose (6 unit equivalent) of platelets in patients taking antiplatelet agents, such as aspirin or clopidogrel, at the time of ICH onset. However, this is controversial.

Seizure Prevention

Although commonly provided, it is not clear that routine antiepileptic (AED) use is beneficial. Seizures are more common in cortical ICH, and, therefore, AED therapy is used in these patients in some centers during the early phase (up to 10 days). AED therapy is indicated in patients who have had a seizure. Agents to consider include:

- Phenytoin 20 mg/kg IV
- Fosphenytoin 20 mg phenytoin equivalents/kg IV
- Valproate 10–15 mg/kg IV
- Levetiracetam 500–1500 mg IV
- Phenobarbital 20 mg/kg IV

Hyperthermia Management

Evaluate for a source of infection, and provide antipyretics as needed.

Hyperglycemia Management

Clinical trials are conflicting on the benefits of intensive insulin therapy; although critically ill patients, in general, benefit from it, it is not clear that those with cerebrovascular emergencies do. However, many patients with ICH have hyperglycemia on presentation, and the higher the glucose, the worse the outcome. Therefore, it is recommended that hyperglycemia (either glucose >185 mg/dl or even glucose >140 mg/dl) be treated with insulin.

Cardiac Monitoring

Cardiac arrhythmias are relatively common after ICH. Patients should be on a cardiac monitor in the acute phase.

Management of Edema or Herniation

Patients with evidence of herniation should receive emergency neurosurgery consultation. Until an intervention can be performed, temporizing measures include:

- Elevation of the head of the bed at 30 degrees with neck in neutral position.
- Ensure that any C-spine collar or other lines or clothing are not constricting venous outflow
- Osmotherapy: Consider
  - Mannitol 20% 0.25–0.5 g/kg.
  - Hypertonic saline. The optimal dosing is not clear. Consider 3% NaCl as a bolus of 250 cc over 20 minutes, or 23.4% NaCl (4 mEq/ml) 30 ml delivered intravenously over 20 minutes.
- Barbiturates: Consider:
  - Pentobarbital 10 mg/kg.
  - Thiopental 1.5–3.5 mg/kg.
- Paralysis: Consider:
  - Vecuronium 0.1 mg/kg.
  - Pancuronium 0.1 mg/kg.
- Hyperventilation (Temporary measure only): Raise the ventilation rate with a constant tidal volume, for a goal pCO_2 25–30 mm^2 Hg.
- External ventricular drain (EVD) placement with ICP monitoring, for a goal ICP <20 mmHg.

Surgery and Endovascular Therapy

Surgery for cerebellar ICH can be life saving and deficit sparing. Emergency neurosurgical consultation is prudent for all patients with cerebellar ICH. The role of surgical hematoma evacuation in supratentorial ICH, on the other hand, remains to be defined. Selected patients with lobar, easily accessible hematomas may be candidates for hematoma evacuation.

ICP Monitoring and EVD Placement

ICP monitoring should be considered for patients with clinical or radiographic evidence of hydrocephalus, or for patients in whom therapies aimed at decreasing ICP will be used. Consider EVD placement for patients with intraventricular blood who show signs of or are at risk of developing hydrocephalus. In addition, some may consider patients with intraventricular hemorrhage for experimental or off-label intervention involving application of thrombolytics through indwelling intraventricular catheters.

Prediction of Outcome

Although not usually addressed in the first hours of care, one of the major challenges facing providers and families is providing accurate information about likely outcome. Decisions regarding surgical intervention, Do Not Resuscitate (DNR) orders, inter-hospital transfer, and allocation of scarce resources must often take into account expected outcomes. Because ICH is a devastating event, decisions to withdraw aggressive care can become a self-fulfilling prophecy; as a result, the American Heart Association recommends that no DNR order be placed in the first 24 hours. A formal scoring system should be considered when offering prognostic information. The FUNC score[14], see Figure 4.3, can be used to predict likelihood of return to independent functional status.

Secondary ICH Management

ICH can be secondary to a number of causes. ICH secondary to trauma is addressed in another chapter (Chapter 9) as is that secondary to hemorrhagic conversion of an ischemic infarct (Chapter 3). Other causes are outlined in the following sections.

Arteriovenous Malformations

The natural history of acute bleeding secondary to an arteriovenous malformation (AVM) is less well studied than that of primary ICH. The American Heart Association does offer formal guidelines. The most important intervention is emergent consultation with an interventional neurologist, an interventional neuroradiologist, or a neurosurgeon. Typically, there is little indication for emergent surgery except to release the mass effect of the hematoma.

- Options for securing the AVM include:
  - Surgical excision.
  - Endovascular techniques such as embolization.
  - Radiosurgery.
  - A combination of the preceding three modalities.
- Medical management: The degree to which patients with AVM-related ICH are at risk for hematoma expansion is unknown. Typically the guidelines of blood pressure management and

Determination of the ICH Score	
Component	**ICH Score Points**
GCS score	
3–4	2
5–12	1
13–15	0
ICH volume, cm³	
≥30	1
<30	0
IVH	
Yes	1
No	0
Infratentorial origin of ICH	
Yes	1
No	0
Age, y	
≥80	1
<80	0
Total ICH Score	0–6

GCS score indicates GCS score on initial presentation (or after resuscitation); ICH volume, volume on the initial CT calculated using *ABC*/2 method; and IVH, presence of any IVH on initial CT.

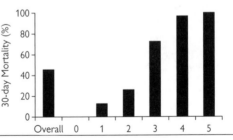

Figure 4.3 FUNC score determination and related mortality

anticoagulation reversal prescribed for primary ICH are followed in cases of AVM-related ICH.

Aneurysmal Subarachnoid Hemorrhage (SAH)

The classic history is one of a thunderclap headache, with or without neurological signs. Importantly, about 30–40 percent of SAH

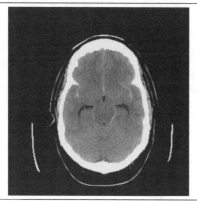

Figure 4.4 CT scan showing subarachnoid hemorrhage.

patients will not have focal neurological symptoms or signs. Once SAH is diagnosed (see Figure 4.4), consult with an interventional team that includes vascular neurosurgery and interventional neurology/neuroradiology. The American Heart Association offers guidelines for the care of aneurysmal SAH, which are incorporated here. Differential diagnosis of thunderclap headache:

- Aneurysmal SAH
- Perimesencephalic SAH
- Benign thunderclap headache
- Pituitary apoplexy
- Cerebral venous sinus thrombosis
- Cranio-cephalic arterial dissection
- Hypertensive encephalopathy

To establish the underlying vascular lesion, vascular imaging is critical.

- DSA: This study is traditionally the gold standard for visualization and preoperative planning. MRA and CTA can be considered when DSA cannot be performed in a timely fashion or if the specialist can do the procedure based on the noninvasive imaging alone.
- CTA: Widely available, often provides a clear view of the vasculature, and is used in some centers as the only modality for surgical planning.
- MRA: Advantages include use of MRI to evaluate alternative causes of bleeding, and that MRA can be performed without contrast in those patients at risk for nephrotoxicity.

Disadvantages include speed of image acquisition, less availability, and problems with contraindications.

- In approximately 15 percent of patients with nontraumatic subarachnoid hemorrhage, no aneurysm is found. It is not clear whether these patients have aneurysms too small to be detected with available technology, or have bleeding from a nonaneurysmal source. For patients in whom the subarachnoid blood accumulates exclusively in what is known as a perimesencephalic pattern, good outcome is generally the rule, and complications such as the development of secondary cerebral injury from vasospasm are very uncommon.

SAH Management

Emergently secure the aneurysm

The cornerstone of therapy is endovascular coiling or surgical clipping, which should be performed as early as possible to reduce the risk of rebleeding. Referral to high volume centers with both cerebrovascular surgeons and endovascular specialists is associated with improved outcomes.

Supportive Care

Medical management is similar to ICH management already discussed. Airway management, cardiac monitoring, hyperglycemia management, and anticoagulation reversal should be performed as discussed in the preceding section. Issues specific to SAH are as follows.

Blood Pressure Management

There are no specific AHA recommendations. Many centers use pharmacotherapy emergently to lower SBP below 140, which may minimize risk of aneurysmal re-rupture. Recommended agents include:

- Labetalol: Intermittent boluses of 10–40 mg, or continuous drop (2–8 mg/min)
- Esmolol: 500 mcg/kg load, then 50–200 mcg/kg/min maintenance
- Nicardipine: 5–15 mg/hour
- Increasingly, experts are recommending the avoidance of nitroprusside

Antifibrinolytic Therapy

This approach may be considered, although its use is becoming less common as more centers perform emergent interventions to secure the aneurysm. The AHA suggests this approach can be used as follows:

- With a short course, combined with early securing of the aneurysm followed by discontinuation of the antifibrinolytic and prophylaxis against hypovolemia and vasospasm.

86

- In certain clinical situations, in conjunction with the interventional team, for example, for those with a low risk of vasospasm or with a benefit expected from delayed surgery.
- Agents have included epsilon aminocaproic acid (36 g/d) or tranexamic acid (6–12 g/d).

Prevention of Vasospasm and Delayed Cerebral Ischemia

- Nimodipine should be provided as early as possible (60 mg orally or per NG tube, every 4 hours) for a duration of 21 days.
- Avoid hypovolemia.
- Use of volume expansion, induced hypertension, and hemodilution (triple-H) should be considered in patients with symptomatic cerebral vasospasm but is generally avoided until after the aneurysm is secured.
- Cerebral angioplasty and/or intra-arterial vasodilator therapy can be reasonable.

Treatment of Hydrocephalus

Patients with hydrocephalus are candidates for emergency EVD placement.

Seizure Management

There is no clear benefit to prophylactic anti-epileptic drug (AED) therapy in the absence of known seizures. Prophylactic AEDs can be considered in the acute phase. Some data suggest that phenytoin, in particular, may worsen outcome. The only clear indication for AED therapy is in those patients who have had a seizure (see the seizure prevention section above for common AED choices).

Cerebral Venous Sinus Thrombosis (CVST)

These patients often have headache with or without associated focal neurologic signs and symptoms. As a result, the diagnosis of ICH secondary to CVST can be difficult and requires a high degree of suspicion.

- The presence of headache, papilledema or other signs of increased ICP, seizures at presentation, absence of classical risk factors for ischemic stroke, relatively young age, and history of ulcerative colitis should serve as red flags.
- Radiologic findings that can raise suspicion include:
  - Hyperdense cerebral veins, a "delta sign" on noncontrast CT scan (a dense triangle within the superior sagittal sinus).
  - Presence of underlying infarction in a nonarterial distribution.
  - Presence of multiple hemorrhages.

Use of contrast-enhanced neuroimaging, such as MR venography or CT venography, may be necessary for diagnosis.

Management is directed at arresting clot propagation and the development of cerebral venous infarction, cerebral edema, and brain herniation. A set of European guidelines are available, which are summarized here.

Supportive care should be as has been discussed earlier for ICH, including airway management, hyperglycemia management, seizure prophylaxis, and ICP management.

Anticoagulation

Dose adjusted intravenous unfractionated heparin (for a goal of at least doubling the partial thromboplastin time) should be considered in patients without contraindications. It is important to note that the presence of ICH in patients with CVST is not considered an absolute contraindication to anticoagulation.

Thrombolysis

Intrasinus thromborrhexis and thrombolysis are performed in experienced centers and should be considered in patients in whom restoration of venous drainage is expected to be life saving and/or deficit sparing.

Suggested Reading

Anderson CS, Huang Y, Wang JG, et al. Intensive blood pressure reduction in acute cerebral haemorrhage trial (INTERACT): a randomised pilot trial. *Lancet Neurol.* 2008;7:391–399.

Bederson JB, Connolly ES, Jr., Batjer HH, et al. Guidelines for the management of aneurysmal subarachnoid hemorrhage: a statement for healthcare professionals from a special writing group of the Stroke Council, American Heart Association. *Stroke.* 2009;40:994–1025.

Broderick J, Connolly S, Feldmann E, et al. Guidelines for the management of spontaneous intracerebral hemorrhage in adults: 2007 update: a guideline from the American Heart Association/American Stroke Association Stroke Council, High Blood Pressure Research Council, and the Quality of Care and Outcomes in Research Interdisciplinary Working Group. *Stroke.* 2007;38:2001–2023.

Delgado Almandoz JE, Schaefer PW, Forero NP, Falla JR, Gonzalez RG, Romero JM. Diagnostic accuracy and yield of multidetector ct angiography in the evaluation of spontaneous intraparenchymal cerebral hemorrhage. *AJNR Am J Neuroradiol.* 2009.

Einhaupl K, Bousser MG, de Bruijn SF, Ferro JM, Martinelli I, Masuhr F, Stam J. EFNS guideline on the treatment of cerebral venous and sinus thrombosis. *Eur J Neurol.* 2006;13:553–559.

Flibotte JJ, Hagan N, O'Donnell J, Greenberg SM, Rosand J. Warfarin, hematoma expansion, and outcome of intracerebral hemorrhage. *Neurology.* 2004; 63:1059–1064.

Gray CS, Hildreth AJ, Sandercock PA, et al. Glucose-potassium-insulin infusions in the management of post-stroke hyperglycaemia: the UK Glucose Insulin in Stroke Trial (GIST-UK). *Lancet Neurol.* 2007;6:397–406.

Hemphill JC, 3rd, Newman J, Zhao S, Johnston SC. Hospital usage of early do-not-resuscitate orders and outcome after intracerebral hemorrhage. *Stroke.* 2004;35:1130–1134.

Hemphill JC, 3rd, Bonovich DC, Besmertis L, Manley GT, Johnston SC. The ICH score: a simple, reliable grading scale for intracerebral hemorrhage. *Stroke.* 2001;32:891–897.

Mayer SA, Brun NC, Begtrup K, et al. Efficacy and safety of recombinant activated factor VII for acute intracerebral hemorrhage. *N Engl J Med.* 2008;358:2127–2137.

Meredith W, Rutledge R, Fakhry SM, Emery S, Kromhout-Schiro S. The conundrum of the Glasgow Coma Scale in intubated patients: a linear regression prediction of the Glasgow verbal score from the Glasgow eye and motor scores. *J Trauma.* 1998;44:839–844; discussion 844–835.

Naff NJ, Hanley DF, Keyl PM, et al. Intraventricular thrombolysis speeds blood clot resolution: results of a pilot, prospective, randomized, double-blind, controlled trial. *Neurosurgery.* 2004;54:577–583; discussion 583–574.

Ogilvy CS, Stieg PE, Awad I, et al. AHA Scientific Statement: Recommendations for the management of intracranial arteriovenous malformations: a statement for healthcare professionals from a special writing group of the Stroke Council, American Stroke Association. *Stroke.* 2001;32:1458–1471.

Rost NS, Smith EE, Chang Y, et al. Prediction of functional outcome in patients with primary intracerebral hemorrhage: the FUNC score. *Stroke.* 2008;39:2304–2309.

Smith EE, Rosand J, Greenberg SM. Imaging of hemorrhagic stroke. *Magn Reson Imaging Clin N Am.* 2006;14:127140.

Steiner T, Kaste M, Forsting M, et al. Recommendations for the management of intracranial haemorrhage—part I: spontaneous intracerebral haemorrhage. The European Stroke Initiative Writing Committee and the Writing Committee for the EUSI Executive Committee. *Cerebrovasc Dis.* 2006;22:294–316.

Van den Berghe G, Wilmer A, Hermans G, et al. Intensive insulin therapy in the medical ICU. *N Engl J Med.* 2006;354:449–461.

Walls RM, Murphy MF, et al. *Manual of Emergency Airway Management* Philadelphia: Lippincott Williams & Wilkins; 2004.

Chapter 5

Seizures

Michael Ganetsky and Frank W. Drislane

Isolated Seizures

An epileptic seizure is a paroxysmal burst of abnormal and excessively synchronized neuronal activity causing a clinical neurologic deficit with signs or symptoms. A seizure usually has a clear, abrupt onset and a discernible (but often less discrete) ending, and may be followed by a postictal phase that involves lethargy or confusion. The symptoms and signs vary from one patient to the next but are stereotypic for an individual patient, according to the brain area involved. They can be sensory, motor, autonomic, or cognitive in nature.

A seizure may be unprovoked or it may be provoked by medication use, medication withdrawal, sleep deprivation or disturbance, trauma, stroke, metabolic disturbance, infection, or toxins. A seizure may be accompanied by an 'aura,' such as a stereotyped sensation (e.g., olfactory hallucination) while awareness is still intact; this is the beginning of the seizure, but awareness is maintained such that the patient can still report the sensation.

First Seizure

After a first unprovoked seizure, the risk of recurrence over the next few years is about 45 percent for seizures in general, with treatment, and slightly greater without treatment (most of these data were obtained in children). A first unprovoked seizure is defined as one occurring in a person over one month of age with no earlier seizure (excluding neonatal and febrile seizures) and not due to some provocation such as head trauma, infection, stroke, metabolic derangement, or toxin. The recurrence rate is influenced strongly by the cause of the seizure. Rates are higher for patients with an abnormal EEG, a structural CNS lesion, presentation with status epilepticus or febrile seizures, or with a family history of epilepsy.

Seizure Classification

- A simple partial (or focal) seizure involves part of the brain and does not impair consciousness.
- Complex partial seizures are of focal onset but associated with impaired consciousness, which may occur at the start of the seizure or develop later. Complex partial seizures often present as "spells" of altered response or behavior; they may include automatisms, but not convulsions.
- Generalized seizures have symptoms consistent with involvement of a large area of both hemispheres. Generalized 'tonic-clonic' seizures include (often violent) tonic, then clonic, motor activity, and loss of consciousness.
- Absence seizures are also generalized. They present with impaired consciousness, but essentially no motor activity.

Evaluation of a First Isolated Seizure

The evaluation of the first seizure is outlined in the bulleted points that follow, but the studies need not all be done in the emergency department. For patients who live with a responsible adult and are reliable in follow-up, and who have had a nonfocal seizure and a rapid return of normal mental status, most of the work-up can be done in the outpatient setting. Still, in the ED, most physicians will obtain a head CT, basic blood work, and an EKG, as these are readily available and can screen for ominous illnesses. A first focal seizure warrants a more urgent work-up, given the concern for a structural CNS lesion; an MRI with contrast will almost always be necessary at some point.

- Imaging of the brain (CT head or MRI brain).
- CBC, serum chemistry, including sodium, calcium, magnesium and phosphate levels; renal function tests, and a toxicology screen.
- EKG (screen for prolonged QRS or QTc interval).
- Lumbar puncture, if CNS infection suspected.
- EEG (see the last section of this chapter).

Treatment of a First Isolated Seizure

The decision to start an anti-epileptic drug (AED) after a first isolated, *unprovoked* seizure is controversial. An abnormal EEG suggests a higher recurrence risk, but the EEG is rarely obtained in the ED in this circumstance. AED treatment reduces the risk of recurrent seizures in the near future but does not change the long-term prognosis or decrease the risk of developing epilepsy (defined as the tendency to have recurrent unprovoked seizures). Most experts recommend waiting for a second seizure before starting AEDs, as AEDs can have side effects and might be unnecessary. Still, many patients feel safer when they take AEDs, even in this situation, especially if driving or the supervision of children are important activities of daily living. (Of course, driving is allowed only after a seizure-free interval; see next section.) Discussion later with a neurologist is often appropriate. An important part of the history is determining whether this was truly a first seizure. If there were earlier (perhaps less dramatic) seizures, the patient probably has epilepsy already, and AEDs are usually warranted.

Treatment of an isolated *provoked* seizure should be directed at the cause. AED therapy may be avoided if the cause is readily reversible, and unless the seizure was prolonged or a recurrence is likely, for example, with a new CNS mass lesion.

Evaluation and Treatment of an Isolated Seizure in a Patient with Known Epilepsy

- Do a thorough history and physical examination, focused on discovering a precipitating cause (e.g., infection, toxin, sleep deprivation, head injury, missed or new medication, or an intercurrent medical illness).

- Consider serum anti-epileptic drug (AED) concentrations.
- Run CBC, serum chemistry; chest X-ray, and urinalysis, if infection is suspected.
- Get a CT of the head if there are new or changed seizure manifestations or significant head trauma.

The management of a single, isolated seizure in a patient with known epilepsy should include a brief observation period to be sure there is no recurrence. Any precipitating factors should be addressed. If the patient takes an AED that has a (rapidly measurable) concentration that is low, an appropriate dose of that medication should be given to increase the level. If there has been a recent increase in seizure frequency or duration, the patient's neurologist should be contacted to discuss longer observation or changes in management.

NB: Any patient who has had a seizure (or other loss of consciousness) should be informed about local state regulations concerning driving a motor vehicle or operating potentially dangerous machinery. Most states prohibit driving (on or off AEDs) for several months or years after a seizure. This is a legal matter; the physician does not give permission to drive. The clinician should inform the patient (and family) of the local laws and write carefully in the medical record that the discussion took place. Many states require the clinician to report the seizure to the state.

Seizure Mimics

There are many conditions that mimic seizures and should be considered in the differential when evaluating a patient with a history concerning a seizure. Conditions mimicking seizure include:

- Cardiogenic syncope (e.g., from valvular disease, arrhythmias, etc.)
- Vasovagal syncope and autonomic dysfunction
- Convulsive syncope (syncope with a few convulsive jerks)
- Psychogenic nonepileptic seizures (pseudoseizures)
- Gastrointestinal reflux and breath-holding spells in infants
- Movement disorders, such as tics, tremors, choreoathetosis, dystonia
- Transient ischemic attacks
- Transient global amnesia
- Complex migraine
- Myoclonus (e.g., toxin or drug-induced, sleep-related)
- Tetany (e.g., with tetanus, hypocalcemia, strychnine)
- Hypoglycemia

Clinical Pearls

- Patients with TIAs usually have negative symptoms (the absence of movement) rather than positive symptoms (e.g., limb shaking), but remember that complex partial seizures (the most common type in adults) usually occur without motor manifestations and that some patients with high-garde carotid stenosis may present with limb shaking TIAs.
- Many patients with pseudoseizures also have a history of epileptic seizures.
- A minority of patients with otherwise typical vasovagal syncope will have a few clonic jerking movements, especially if they are not allowed to lie supine.

Toxicologic Causes

Many medications, environmental toxins, and withdrawal syndromes can cause seizures or status epilepticus. Some toxins, such as camphor, present with only a brief, isolated seizure, while others, such as isoniazid and tetramine, may lead to status epilepticus refractory to most treatment. The following contains a nonexhaustive list, and specific treatments to toxin-induced seizures are outlined in Table 5.1:

- Sedative/hypnotic withdrawal (ethanol, benzodiazepines, barbiturates) , especially short-acting medications.
- Sympathomimetics (bupropion, cocaine, amphetamines)
- Isoniazid
- Lithium
- Salicilates
- Antidepressants (tricyclics, monoamine oxidase inhibitors, serotonin/norepinephrine reuptake inhibitors, selective serotonin reuptake inhibitors)
- Antibiotics (metronidazole, cephalosporins, penicillins, flouroquinolones).
- Methylxanthines (caffeine, theophylline)
- Carbamazepine, phenytoin (rare, and usually only with very high levels)
- Chloroquine
- Ethylene glycol (from hypocalcemia)
- Synthetic opioids (meperidine, propoxyphene)
- Heavy metals (arsenic, thallium, copper, lead, manganese)
- Household toxins (camphor, fluoride, phenol)
- Pesticides/rodenticides (organophosphates, lindane, pyrethroids, tetramine, zinc phosphide)
- Plant toxins (water hemlock, Ackee fruit, nicotine, false morel)

Table 5.1 Toxin-Induced Seizures with Specific Treatments	
Toxin	Specific Management
Isoniazid Monomethylhydrazine (rocket fuel) Gyromitra mushrooms (false morel)	Pyridoxine 1:1 replacement if ingested dose known; otherwise 5 grams PO/NG/IV
Salycilates Lithium Methylxanthines (theophylline, caffeine)	Seizure is an indication for emergency hemodialysis
TCAs Diphenhydramine Any other agents with sodium channel blockade	NaBicarbonate infusion if QRS is wider than 100 msec
Ethylene glycol	IV calcium (seizures due to hypocalcemia)
Carbon monoxide	Strongly consider hyperbaric oxygen
Cyanide	Hydroxocobalamin or sodium nitrite/sodium thiosulfate
Organophosphates	Diazepam, pralidoxime, atropine
Chloroquine	High dose diazepam, epinephrine
Tetramine (Chinese rodenticide) Cicutoxin (water hemlock)	Refractory GCSE common Consider second and third line AED therapy early in management (see Table 5.2)

- Occupational (monomethylhydrazine, benzene, toluene, hydrogen sulfide, methyl bromide)
- Environmental toxins (carbon monoxide, cyanide)
- Medication-induced mimics: carisoprodol myoclonus, lithium tremor, neuroleptic dystonia, serotonin syndrome
- Environmental mimics (strychnine, tetanus, snake venom fasciculations)

Bupropion, which is indicated for treatment of depression and smoking cessation, is structurally a substitute amphetamine. Depending on the dose, the incidence of seizures with therapeutic dosing is 0.3–0.8 percent and can increase to 33 percent in the setting of overdose. Thus, bupropion is currently a relatively common cause of seizures in patients taking antidepressant medication and should be specifically addressed during the history.

Febrile Seizures

Febrile seizures are the most common cause of seizure in childhood, occurring in about 4 percent of all children. The peak incidence is 18 months, but they can occur from six months to five years of age.

Febrile seizures are thought to be due to the fever directly, and are not, by themselves, signs of a CNS infection. In order to diagnose a febrile seizure, a fever should be present immediately after the seizure. Children with earlier nonfebrile seizures (epilepsy) should not receive this diagnosis.

Febrile seizures are classified as simple (about 70 percent of cases) or complex. Simple febrile seizures are defined in the following section. A complex seizure is one that does not qualify as simple. Complex febrile seizures should be approached in the same way as for a first isolated seizure in an adult, typically requiring neuroimaging and blood work.

Simple Febrile Seizure

- Age six months to five years
- Occurs during a febrile episode
- Generalized (nonfocal) seizure
- Single (does not recur within 24 hours)
- Lasts less than 15 minutes
- No neurologic deficit postictally

The risk of recurrence of a febrile seizure is about 30–40 percent overall, but much lower if the child is older than 18 months, if there is no history of epilepsy or febrile seizures in a first-degree relative, and if the child does not have frequent febrile illnesses. After a simple febrile seizure, the risk of developing epilepsy is only minimally higher than in the general population; it is higher after a complex febrile seizure.

The evaluation of a child with a simple febrile seizure addresses primarily the source of the fever; blood work, EEG, and imaging are almost never necessary, assuming the child has recovered normal neurologic function. The possibility of meningitis (and, if antibiotics have been given, a partially treated meningitis) must be considered. A lumbar puncture (LP) is usually unnecessary if a child over the age of 18 months appears healthy (to a physician familiar with toddlers) after the seizure. LP should be given serious consideration in a child under 12 months of age.

Most clinicians recommend around-the-clock antipyretic therapy for 24 to 48 hours after a febrile seizure, although there is no evidence that this prevents recurrence. Some prescribe rectal diazepam that parents can administer at home if a seizure becomes prolonged (more than three minutes), but this is usually unnecessary as simple febrile seizures typically follow a benign course.

Clinical Pearls

- Remember to consider causes of the seizure other than fever, for example, trauma or toxin.
- After a simple febrile seizure, EEG, neuroimaging and admission are not needed, assuming the child appears healthy overall.

- Lab work should be directed toward addressing the cause of the fever and not the seizure.
- Current recommendations do not include an LP in a child over 18 months old who appears healthy after a simple febrile seizure. LP should be considered in those under a year of age, if meningeal signs are present, or if there are other reasons to suspect a CNS infection.
- AED prophylaxis is not recommended for simple febrile seizures as they are benign and tend to not recur or they remit with age.
- Never attribute a seizure to the fever alone if the patient is older than five years, if there were earlier nonfebrile seizures, or if there are other signs of neurologic illness or systemic illness beyond the infection.

Generalized Convulsive Status Epilepticus

Emergency: Generalized convulsive status epilepticus (GCSE) is a medical and neurologic emergency. Delay in treatment can decrease the likelihood of a good response to treatment and can be followed by persistent neurologic deficits.

Status epilepticus (SE) is defined as a prolonged seizure or recurrent seizures without recovery of consciousness between seizures. What constitutes a prolonged seizure is a matter of debate. The standard definition of status epilepticus includes a duration of 30 minutes, but 5 minutes should be used as a practical, operational guide, because few seizures lasting this long will stop on their own. SE should be differentiated between GCSE and Nonconvulsive Status Epilepticus (NCSE) based on the presence or absence of convulsive motor activity. NCSE is discussed in the next section.

Clinical Pearls

- SE mortality is 17–26 percent in different series, and 10–23 percent of patients who survive are left with neurologic deficits (but mortality and morbidity are almost always due to the underlying cause of SE, e.g., strokes or encephalitis).
- More than 90 percent of generalized tonic-clonic seizures stop after two minutes without treatment and do not become SE.

Etiology of Status Epilepticus

The causes of SE vary with age:

- In children under the age of two, non-CNS infection, fever, and genetic disorders are the most common causes.

- In older children common causes are low levels of AEDs, metabolic disturbances, and may be drug related.
- In adults, common causes include low levels of AEDs, cerebrovascular disease (both ischemic and hemorrhagic), earlier brain injury, metabolic disturbances, alcohol withdrawal, CNS mass, drug ingestion, and trauma.

Management of Generalized Convulsive Status Epilepticus

An overview of management is in Table 5.2.

Treatment of GCSE begins with the ABCs and supportive care:

- Assess airway and breathing; administer supplemental oxygen; place on a cardiac monitor and pulse oximetry, and obtain intravenous access.
- A finger-stick blood glucose should be obtained rapidly, because hypoglycemia can cause SE and seizure activity may be terminated readily with administration of intravenous dextrose.
- The patient's clothes should be removed and a quick exam performed looking for traumatic injuries.
- Any available history from family, paramedics, and other observers should be obtained rapidly.
- Blood, urine, and an EKG should be obtained, and imaging of the CNS should be planned for when the patient is stable.

Next, treatment of any cardiac or metabolic derangement should be addressed:

- A dysrhythmia could have been the cause of an embolic stroke, in turn causing SE (and some dysrhythmias can be caused by seizures), and should be treated per ACLS protocols.
- Hypotension should be treated with intravenous fluids and vasopressors, as needed.
- Fever should be controlled with an antipyretic. If hyperthermia is thought to be from environmental exposure, rapid cooling measures must be instituted. If hyperthermia is thought to be from muscular heat production, endotracheal intubation and pharmacologic paralysis may be considered.
- If the patient has major hyponatremia or hypocalcemia, hypertonic saline or calcium should be administered, respectively.
- If the QRS interval is greater than 100 msec and intoxication with a sodium channel blocking agent (e.g., a TCA) or salicylates is suspected, serum alkalinization should be started with a bicarbonate infusion (3 ampules of Sodium Bicarbonate in 1 liter normal saline infused at 1.5–2 times maintenance).

Table 5.2 Management of Generalized Convulsive Status Epilepticus

Time	Action/Medication	Notes
Arrival	Assess airway and breathing. Provide supplemental oxygen and suction airway. Place on cardiac monitor and pulse oximetry. Establish intravenous access. Disrobe and assess for trauma. Consider immobilizing cervical spine. Obtain any available history. Check FSBG and provide D50W if hypoglycemic.	Hypoventilation, hypoxia, hypoglycemia, dysrhythmias and obvious metabolic derangements should be addressed rapidly. Consider thiamine 100 mg IV prior to D50W if nutritional deficiency suspected.
First 10 minutes	Obtain EKG, blood and urine. Lorazepam 2–4 mg IV (0.1 mg/kg) q 5 minutes. If no IV access: diazepam 20 mg PR or midazolam 10 mg buccally.	In the presence of a wide QRS interval, or if salicylate intoxication suspected, consider bicarbonate infusion.
10–30 minutes	Second line therapy: Phenytoin 20 mg/kg IV at 150 mg/min, or Fosphenytoin 20 mg/kg (PE, phenytoin equivalent) IV at 150 mg/min. Consider pyridoxine 5 gm (by IV or NG tube) if history of isoniazid, gyrometrin mushroom, or hydrazine exposure is suspected. If hypoxia or airway compromise is developing, should perform endotracheal intubation with a short-acting paralytic (such as succynilcholine). At this point, can skip third line agents and move directly to continuous infusion therapy.	If at a location where no continuous EEG or neurologist is available, consider transferring to a tertiary care center. Phenytoin, and most AEDs, can cause hypotension, especially with rapid infusion rates. Fosphenytoin can be infused more rapidly, and causes fewer injection site reactions, compared to phenytoin, but it is more expensive. Once the patient is intubated, avoid long-acting paralysis as this may mask underlying seizure activity.

30–90 minutes	For refractory GCSE (after failure of 2 AEDs): Intubation is necessary at this point. Paralysis is not usually necessary, as the continuous infusion will usually be adequately sedating. Continuous infusion therapy: Pentobarbital 5 mg/kg over 10 min; then continue 1–5 mg/kg/hour, or more, until seizures stop. Propofol 1–2 mg/kg bolus q3–5 minutes until seizures stop, then continue 1–15 mg/kg/hour Midazolam 0.2 mg/kg q5 minutes until seizures stop, then continue 0.1 up to max of 3 mg/kg/hour. • Replete prior AEDs, if low serum levels. • Identify and treat any medical conditions. • Hypertonic saline if severe hyponatremia is present. IV calcium if serious hypocalcemia present.	If using a paralytic agent for rapid sequence intubation, use a short-acting agent. Patient should have bedside consultation by a neurologist and EEG in progress or planned urgently. Continuous AED infusion should be accompanied by continuous EEG monitoring, with the treatment titrated to seizure suppression on the EEG. Acidosis usually resolves when convulsions stop—if it doesn't, look for another cause of acidosis (e.g., toxin, sepsis or propofol infusion syndrome). If sedative/hypnotic withdrawal is suspected and not responding to benzodiazepines, phenobarbital or propofol have shown good results.
30–90 minutes	For NCSE, focal SE, and when intubation is to be avoided: Third line therapy: Phenobarbital 20 mg/kg IV at 75 mg/min Valproate 30 mg/kg IV over 5 minutes Levetiracetam 20 mg/kg IV over 15 minutes Remember to follow initial boluses with maintenance doses	Most patients treated with a combination of a benzodiazepine and a barbiturate will require intubation.

NB: When seizures last more than five minutes, they are unlikely to stop on their own. Response to AEDs declines with time as treatment is delayed. SE often becomes resistant to AEDs with delayed treatment.

After five minutes of continuous seizure activity, treatment with AEDs should be initiated promptly; metabolic derangements should also be addressed.

- Intravenous AED administration is optimal, but rectal diazepam or intramuscular/buccal midazolam are options if IV access is not established.
- Benzodiazepines are considered first-line therapy and will control SE in 80 percent of patients if initiated within 30 minutes. Intravenous lorazepam (0.1 mg/kg) is generally considered the benzodiazepine of choice in SE.
- Pharmacologic paralysis may be necessary for airway control and rapid sequence intubation (RSI). Subsequently, however, such paralysis should seldom be continued because it is NOT a treatment for SE; because AEDs used for SE are usually sufficiently sedating; and because the effectiveness of SE treatment is assessed by the clinical examination—unless continuous EEG is available.

Refractory Status Epilepticus

Refractory SE is defined as seizure activity that persists (clinically or on EEG) despite administration of appropriate doses of two AEDs. Of note, refractoriness is predicted more reliably by response to the first AED than by duration of seizures.

Once SE is determined to be refractory:

- Most neurologists would initiate a continuous intravenous infusion of a medication that is very likely to interrupt SE (e.g., midazolam, pentobarbital, or propofol). This requires endotracheal intubation and mechanical ventilation.
- The infusion should usually be continued for 24 hours after seizures have stopped and then tapered slowly (i.e., for propofol or midazolam, which have very short clinical effect; pentobarbital's clinical activity is much longer, and it may not need to be tapered).
- Third-line therapy can be attempted (e.g., intravenous phenobarbital, valproate, or levetiracetam) if the SE is focal or NCSE, or if there is a strong reason to avoid intubation.

Clinical Pearls

- Do not forget to check a blood glucose and rectal temperature on any patient with a prolonged seizure.

- When a seizure lasts more than five minutes, it is unlikely to stop on its own, and AED therapy should be instituted promptly, treating as if the patient has GCSE.
- Prolonged febrile seizures are the most common cause of GCSE in children and should be managed in a manner similar to that for adults.
- Consider a toxicologic cause of seizure in the differential, and consider pyridoxine 5 grams (IV/PO/NG) for any patient (especially children) who does not respond to first-line AEDs.
- Patients with GCSE who are pharmacologically paralyzed may still be seizing even though the peripheral muscle activity is blocked. Such patients need urgent EEG monitoring. Most paralytics used for RSI should clear in 10–15 minutes; further doses should not be given routinely because these patients will usually be adequately sedated by the AEDs. A small dose of a quick-acting paralytic may be needed to facilitate brain imaging.
- After the seizures stop, persistent metabolic acidosis may be due to sepsis, toxins or, if propofol is used (especially in children), the propofol infusion syndrome.

Nonconvulsive Status Epilepticus

Nonconvulsive Status Epilepticus (NCSE) is persisting epileptic seizure activity causing a neurologic deficit, but not convulsions. It is most often manifested as confusion, unresponsiveness, or other altered mental status, but can reflect focal or regional seizure activity, with aphasia or other syndromes.

Common presentations of NCSE in the ED are:

- A continuation of a generalized convulsion or GCSE, after the convulsions themselves have stopped, in which case it should be considered continued GCSE, in terms of significance and treatment.
- A patient with earlier epilepsy who presents confused or poorly responsive (but with no recent convulsions).

NCSE should be considered in any patient who has had a generalized seizure or GCSE whose mental status does not improve within 20 minutes or normalize completely within 60 minutes after convulsions stop. NCSE without earlier motor activity is much harder to diagnose and should be in the differential of altered mental status. For example, NCSE was found in 8 percent of comatose ICU patients without any earlier motor manifestations of seizures.

NCSE is a broad term that includes the following syndromes:

- Continuation of GCSE (see previous paragraph) that has progressed to a dissociation between motor activity and continued electrical seizure activity (i.e., a late stage of GCSE).
- SE in critically ill or comatose patients (often similar to patients in the preceding situation, but sometimes without earlier clinically evident seizures).
- Absence SE, usually in patients with earlier absence seizures.
- Complex partial SE, i.e., focal onset seizures that persist as altered or diminished consciousness.

NCSE can be due to a primary seizure disorder but is more often caused by an acute medical illness (e.g., infectious, metabolic, drug-related). In the elderly, its presentation can be highly variable and may include personality changes, confusion, psychosis, and rarely, coma. NCSE is also relatively common in critically ill children, though it is often unrecognized.

Diagnosis

- If NCSE is being considered, urgent electroencephalogram (EEG) should be performed.
- NCSE should be suspected if a clear clinical improvement occurs quickly after administration of an AED. Because of their rapid onset of effect, benzodiazepines are the most commonly used test agents in this situation.
- Patients with NCSE may show subtle motor activity, such as frequent blinking, spontaneous nystagmus, mouth movements, or myoclonic jerks.
- NCSE is diagnosed by characteristic patterns of epileptic seizures on EEG (see Figures 5.1 and 5.2).

Management

GCSE may cause neuronal damage, but NCSE is much less likely to do so. NCSE has many forms, and the prognosis and urgency of treatment vary. Patients with NCSE are sick and need treatment, but aggressive use of AEDs can cause complications. Because treatment of NCSE is controversial and complex, it should be guided by continuous EEG monitoring and with neurologic consultation in the ICU.

- Second-line therapy includes intravenous phenobarbital, phenytoin, fosphenytoin, valproate, and levetiracetam.
- In many cases of NCSE, intravenous (and occasionally oral) benzodiazepines are first-line therapy and may be sufficient.
- Nondisabling focal SE may sometimes be treated less urgently, with oral AEDs, especially those the patient was taking already.

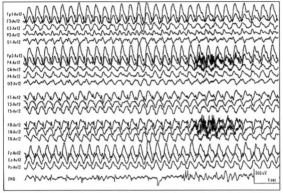

Figure 5.1 Rhythmic 3 Hz spike and slow wave discharges characteristic of absence seizures, or if longer, absence SE. From a 42-year-old woman with earlier juvenile myoclonic epilepsy, presenting with confusion and slowed speech. This NCSE is usually easy to treat.
Source: With permission from Kaplan PW, Drislane FW eds. The electroencephalogram of nonconvulsive status epilepticus. In: *Nonconvulsive Status Epilepticus*. New York: Demos Medical Publishing, 2009:49.

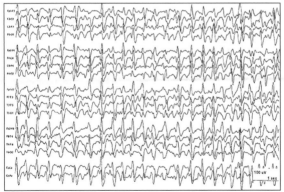

Figure 5.2 Persisting epileptiform discharges of NCSE in a 75-year-old woman with a history of convulsions, now confused and lethargic. The presence of NCSE cannot be determined without EEG, and EEG helps to determine when treatment is successful.
Source: With permission from Kaplan PW, Drislane FW, eds. The electroencephalogram of nonconvulsive status epilepticus. In: *Nonconvulsive Status Epilepticus*. New York: Demos Medical Publishing, 2009:44.

- The NCSE that follows generalized convulsions or GCSE should be considered a continuation of GCSE and treated urgently. Many of these cases become refractory SE.
- NCSE associated with strokes and coma carries a poor prognosis (mostly because of the underlying stroke) and warrants aggressive treatment.

NCSE in comatose patients can be very difficult to diagnose and complicated to manage. Some EEGs show clear seizure patterns, and others are more equivocal. Many patients are in the ICU, with significant metabolic or infectious illnesses. Usually, the underlying critical illness causes the seizures, and it must be dealt with. Also, it is not always clear whether the NCSE causes the coma. In cases of NCSE in the setting of anoxic coma, for example, treatment of seizures seldom leads to improvement because of the severe anoxic damage; in this case, AEDs do not appear to improve outcome.

Clinical Pearls

- Remember to keep NCSE on the differential for any patient with unexplained coma or altered consciousness, especially if there was an earlier seizure.
- Obtain urgent EEG and involve a neurologist to help guide treatment if NCSE is suspected.

Electroencephalography

Epileptic seizures are a clinical diagnosis, made primarily from the history of symptoms by the patient, plus characterization of the event by observers, often the family. When the diagnosis is difficult (e.g., distinguishing in some cases between epileptic seizure and cardiac syncope), the finding of characteristic epileptiform discharges on an EEG can help secure a diagnosis. Nevertheless, about half of patients with epilepsy have normal EEGs at a given time, and finding nonspecific abnormalities is not useful diagnostically. A minority of patients with epilepsy has clear epileptiform abnormalities on EEG. They may be more evident shortly after a seizure (especially in children) so it is best if the EEG is done soon.

Once diagnosis of an epileptic seizure is made, an EEG is appropriate mostly to determine the type of seizure (e.g., focal or generalized in origin) and whether it is part of a recognized epilepsy syndrome, with characteristic EEG discharges and other findings (e.g., temporal lobe epilepsy or absence seizures of adolescence). An EEG characteristic of a particular epilepsy syndrome assists in directing further workup, in the choice of AED, and with prognosis. Neither the EEG to diagnose seizures nor an EEG to help identify an epilepsy syndrome need be done in the ED.

The primary use of EEG in the ED is for the recognition of nonconvulsive status epilepticus. The most common (and threatening) setting is that of a patient who has had a generalized convulsion or GCSE and has not returned to normal function. It is impossible to tell without EEG whether the patient is postictal or in NCSE. Also, a patient presenting with altered mental status can be in NCSE without having had a convulsion, particularly if there was an earlier diagnosis of epilepsy or if the patient has a serious medical illness.

Finally, after diagnosis of SE, the EEG is crucial in guiding treatment, to determine whether the AEDs have stopped the SE, in looking for recurrence of seizures or SE, and in determining how "deeply" seizures are suppressed (the last of these usually occurs in the ICU after the patient has left the ED).

When a patient recovers quickly from seizures or SE, an EEG is not urgent. When the patient has not recovered or the cause of altered mental status has not been determined definitively, the EEG is mandatory.

Suggested Reading

Barry E, Hauser W. Status epilepticus: the interaction of epilepsy and acute brain disease. *Neurology.* 1993;43:1473–1478.

Chen JW, Westerlain CG. Status epilepticus: pathophysiology and management in adults. *Lancet Neurol.* 2006;5:246.

Holtkamp M, Othman J, Buchheim K, Meierkord H. Diagnosis of psychogenic nonpileptic status epilepticus in the emergency setting. *Neurology.* 2006;66:1727–1729.

Husain AM, Horn GJ, Jacobson MP. Non-convulsive status epilepticus: usefulness of clinical features in selecting patients for urgent EEG. *J Neurol Neurosurg Psychiatry.* 2003;74:189–191.

Kaplan PW. Nonconvulsive status epilepticus in the emergency room. *Epilepsia.* 1996;37:643–650.

Kaplan PW, Drislane FW. *Nonconvulsive Status Epilepticus.* New York: Demos Medical Publishing; 2008.

Meierkord H, Holtkamp M. Non-convulsive status epilepticus in adults: clinical forms and treatment. *Lancet Neurol.* 2007;6:329–339.

Shorvon S, Baulac M, Cross H, Trinka E, Walker M; TaskForce on Status Epilepticus of the ILAE Commission for European Affairs. The drug treatment of status epilepticus in Europe: consensus document from a workshop at the first London Colloquium on Status Epilepticus. *Epilepsia.* 2008;49:1277–1284.

Walker M. Status epilepticus: an evidence based guide. *BMJ.* 2005;331:673–677.

Chapter 6

Generalized Weakness

Carl A. Germann and Nicholas J. Silvestri

Introduction

Acute generalized weakness can occur as a result of injury to either the central or peripheral nervous system. This chapter will review generalized weakness that is due to dysfunction of the peripheral nervous system, including diseases of the peripheral nerve, neuromuscular junction, and muscle. Essential spinal cord disorders that may cause weakness will also be described.

A peripheral neuropathy is defined as a dysfunction of motor, sensory, or autonomic nerves, and may involve the entire nerve or discrete segments. A neuromuscular junction (NMJ) disorder affects the synapse of the axon terminal of a motor neuron with the motor endplate, and thus disrupts the initiation of action potentials across the muscle's surface, preventing muscle contraction. A myopathy results in muscular weakness due to dysfunction of the muscle fibers themselves or of ion channels on the muscle membrane, leading to impaired contraction. Though the spinal cord is part of the central nervous system, diseases of the cord (myelopathy) may lead to generalized weakness, occurring from an extradural, intradural extramedullary, or an intramedullary lesion.

Clinically, weakness should first be differentiated into central and peripheral disease. Unlike peripheral processes, CNS disorders often contain signs of cortical disease, such as dysphagia, dysarthria, or lateralization of weakness. In addition, signs and symptoms of upper and lower motor neuron tracts can be helpful in distinguishing a central from a peripheral process. Upper motor neurons originate in the cerebral cortex and terminate in the brainstem or spinal cord. Lower motor neurons originate in the spinal cord (cranial nerves being the exception) and terminate at the neuromuscular junction. The signs of upper motor neuron (UMN) disease include spasticity and hyperreflexia, whereas lower motor neuron (LMN) disease may present with hypotonia and hyporeflexa, and an absence of a Babinksi sign. Notably, an acute UMN lesion may initially present with spinal shock and associated flaccid paralysis while typical signs of a UMN lesion develop later. Located beyond the lower motor neuron tract, patients with neuromuscular junction diseases and myopathies may have normal muscle tone and reflexes. These entities often present with diffuse weakness. Neuromuscular junction diseases commonly involve weakness of the bulbar and respiratory musculature. As opposed to neuropathies, in myopathies the proximal muscles tend to be involved more than distal ones. In diseases of the spinal cord, such as transverse myelitis and spinal cord infarction, both upper and lower neuron symptoms may be present and depend upon the level and extent of the spinal cord involvement (Figure 6.1).

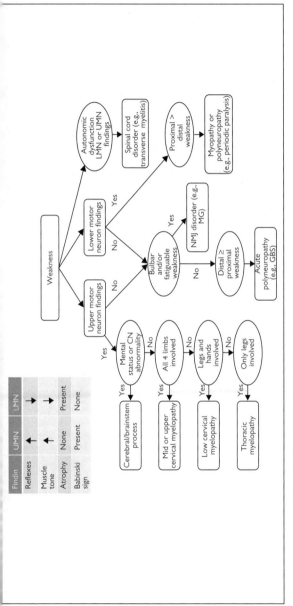

Figure 6.1 Diagnostic algorithm based upon the distribution of weakness.

The clinical progression of weakness and associated symptoms are also helpful in focusing a differential diagnosis. Essential historical features that should be obtained include the time of onset, progression, exacerbating and relieving factors, preceding and associated symptoms, and a prior history of similar problems. In general, peripheral diseases follow a progressive deterioration, whereas central lesions more commonly present in an acute or subacute fashion.

Etiologies

Key emergency conditions selected from this comprehensive list are discussed in more detail in the remainder of the chapter.

Box 6.1 Differential Diagnosis of Acute Weakness

Peripheral Nerve Disorders (Neuropathies)

Toxic Neuropathies
  Heavy metals (arsenic, lead, thallium)
  Drugs (amiodarone, vincristine, dapsone)
  Organophosphates
  Ethanol

Infectious Neuropathies
  Diphtheria
  HIV
  CMV
  Lyme disease

Other Neuropathies (Causing Weakness)
  Guillain Barré syndrome (AIDP)
  Thiamine deficiency
  Hypothyroidism
  Diabetes
  Uremia
  Nutritional (B vitamins)
  Critical illlness polyneuropathy

Neuromuscular Junction Disorders

Myasthenia gravis

Eaton-Lambert syndrome

Botulism

Tick paralysis

Insect/marine toxins

Box 6.1 (Continued)

Myopathies

Polymyositis

Dermatomyositis

Inclusion body myositis

Periodic Paralysis (Hyper- or Hypokalemic)

Alcoholic Myopathy

Drugs (steroids, cholesterol-lowering drugs, AZT)

Spinal Cord Disorders

Transverse myelitis

Syringomyelia

Multiple sclerosis

HIV myelopathy

Dorsal column disorders (syphilis, B12 deficiency)

Tetanus

Spinal cord infarction

Spinal cord compression

Other causes of weakness

Amyotrophic Lateral Sclerosis

Poliomyelitis

Porphyria

113

Neuropathies

Guillain Barré Syndrome

Guillain Barré Syndrome (GBS), also known as acute inflammatory demyelinating polyradiculoneuropathy (AIDP), represents the most common form of acute generalized neuropathy and may affect patients of all ages. Most cases are thought to be due to an autoimmune attack on myelinated motor nerves that is precipitated by an antecedent infection. The most frequently identified causes of preceding infection are Camplyobacter jejuni, cytomegalovirus, Epstein-Barr virus, Mycoplasma pneumonia, and Haemophilus influenza. Vaccinations are another rare cause of GBS. In approximately one-third of cases, an antecedent immunological trigger is not identified.

Presentation

• Patients often present days to weeks after the resolution of a respiratory or gastrointestinal illness.

- The most common symptom is progressive symmetrical weakness of the limbs, involving both proximal and distal muscles.
- Symptoms are typically worse in the lower extremities.
- Initial symptoms may also include low back pain due to involvement of the nerve roots.
- Symptoms may also include paraesthesia of the limbs or gait imbalance due to involvement of large diameter sensory fibers. These sensory symptoms often precede motor symptoms and may rarely occur without associated motor findings.
- GBS is associated with a lack of deep tendon reflexes.
- Fluctuations in pulse and blood pressure (autonomic instability) occurs in approximately two-thirds of patients.
- Respiratory failure is common with one-third of patients requiring ventilator support
- The Miller-Fisher variant of GBS is a triad of ophthalmoplegia, ataxia, and areflexia. Some degree of muscle weakness is usually also present. This syndrome has been associated with the presence of anti-GQ1b antibodies in the serum. This variant may resemble a brainstem process (e.g., stroke) and consideration to urgent imaging of the brain should be given, especially in those with vascular risk factors.
- Another rare variant of GBS is known as polyneuritis cranialis. This is usually seen in younger patients with antecedent CMV infection, and presents with multiple cranial nerve palsies, particularly bilateral seventh nerve involvement. Dysphagia and dysarthia are also common symptoms.

Clinical Pearls

- About two-thirds of patients report symptoms of an infection within three weeks before the onset of GBS symptoms.
- Involvement of sensory fibers may lead to reduction in vibratory sensation and proprioception (joint position sense).
- The clinical signs, degree of symptoms, and timing of disease progression and resolution are highly variable.
- Recurrence rate of GBS is approximately 3 percent.
- Mortality rate is approximately 3–10 percent and most often due to respiratory or autonomic dysfunction.
- The CSF profile may be normal in the first week of symptoms.
- The decision for intubation in patients presenting with GBS is made on a case-by-case basis. As in other neuromuscular disorders with potential diaphragmatic weakness, signs of impending respiratory collapse include tachypnea, use of accessory muscles of inspiration, negative inspiratory force (NIF) less than 20 or forced vital capacity (FVC) less than 15 cc/kg and

are potential indicators for the need for intubation and artificial ventilation. These latter parameters may be artificially low if there is profound facial weakness and inability to form a seal around the instrument used to measure them. Inability to clear secretions and the resultant risk for aspiration is another indication for intubation, as is profound limb weakness which usually heralds respiratory involvement.

Box 6.2 Factors Suggesting Need for Endotracheal Intubation in GBS Patients

- FVC < 15 cc/kg
- NIF < - 20
- Inability to clear secretions (concern for aspiration)
- Use of accessory muscles for breathing

Investigations

- Lumbar puncture should be performed in those suspected of having GBS.
- Cerebrospinal fluid (CSF) protein concentrations are often normal in the first week, but increase in more than 90 percent of patients by the end of the second week of illness.
- An increased pleocytosis should raise the possibility of another illness, such as leptomeningeal infection, Lyme disease, West Nile virus infection, HIV-related GBS, or poliomyelitis.
- As mentioned earlier, bedside pulmonary function tests (PFTs), including NIF and FVC, should be performed once the diagnosis is entertained. A NIF of less than 20 or an FVC less than 15 cc/kg are potential indicators for the need for intubation and artificial ventilation. A consistent downward trend of these parameters over time may also be a sign of impending respiratory collapse.
- Spinal shock due to cord compression or inflammation may also present with limb weakness and areflexia. Any patient suspected of having spinal cord dysfunction (discussed in a separate section later) should have urgent imaging of the spine, preferably MRI.
- Although not typically done emergently, electromyography (EMG) and nerve conduction studies (NCS) may be helpful in clarifying the diagnosis if it is in question. Electrodiagnostic studies are abnormal in about 90 percent of patients within the first five weeks after presentation, though a significant percentage will have some evidence of demyelination on NCS in the first week or two.

Management

- Intravenous immunoglobulin (IVIg) and plasma exchange are effective treatments.
- Patients require regular monitoring for potential pulmonary and autonomic dysfunction.
- Patients that should be admitted to an ICU setting (as opposed to a floor) are those with respiratory compromise (or the potential for imminent respiratory compromise as discussed earlier), those with evidence of autonomic dysfunction, and those with profound limb weakness. Patients without these findings and those that are able to ambulate unassisted are usually appropriate for a floor setting. The pace of the progression of a given patient's symptoms and the monitoring capabilities at any given hospital should also be considered in this decision.

Toxic Neuropathies

Many toxic agents can produce a peripheral neuropathy. Heavy metals, drugs, industrial solvents, organophosphates, and ethanol are among the most common causes of toxic neuropathies. Many neurotoxicities are temporary and resolve as the drug or toxin is removed.

Box 6.3 Toxins

Organic and industrial agents

- Acryamide
- Allyl chloride
- Carbon disulfide
- Ethylene oxide
- Hexacarbons
- Methyl bromide
- Organophosphates
- Polychlorinated biphenyls
- Trichloroethylene
- Vacor

Metals

- Arsenic
- Lead
- Gold
- Mercury
- Thallium

Box 6.3 (Continued)

Therapeutic agents

- Amiodarone
- Antiretrovirals
- Dapsone
- Disulfiram
- Isoniazid
- Metronidazole
- Nitrofurantoin
- Paclitaxel (Taxol)
- Phenytoin
- Statins (Simvastatin, Lovastatin, Pravastatin)
- Vincristine
- Platinum-containing drugs (cisplatin, carboplatin, oxaliplatin)
- Hydralazine
- Linezolid
- Pyridoxine

Clinical Pearls

- Organophosphates are anticholinesterase agents that increase postsynaptic acetylcholine and, therefore, produce procholinergic symptoms.
- Chronic alcohol use can produce a stocking-glove sensory neuropathy.
- Arsenic can also produce a stocking-glove neuropathy that is initially sensory with motor symptoms developing later.
- Lead toxicity can cause paresthesias, motor weakness (wrist drop), depressed DTRs, with intact sensory function.
- It is estimated that 60 percent patients receiving neurotoxic chemotherapeutic agent have some degree of neuropathy

Box 6.4 A Problem Commonly Misdiagnosed

Porphyias are commonly misdiagnosed because patients often present with vague or nonspecific symptoms. Acute intermittent porphyria is an autosomal dominantly inherited disorder of heme synthesis, which may lead to episodes of weakness (primarily proximal limb weakness, but cranial nerve and respiratory involvement may also occur) due to build-up of toxic compounds. Neurologic manifestations are usually accompanied by abdominal pain, psychiatric disturbances, and reddish urine.

Neuromuscular Junction Disorders

Myasthenia Gravis

Myasthenia Gravis is an autoimmune disease caused by acetylcholine (ACh) receptor antibodies at the neuromuscular junction. Impaired receptor function (failure to respond to acetylcholine stimulation) leads to a decrease in muscle fiber potential amplitudes causing diminished muscle strength. This autoimmune response is believed to be due to either a dysfunction in the thymus gland or a result of an immune response to exogenous infectious antigens.

Presentation

- The most common age of onset for females is in the second and third decades.
- The most common age of onset for males is in the seventh and eighth decades.
- The mean duration between symptom onset and diagnosis is one year.
- Common symptoms include ptosis, diplopia, limb weakness, dysphagia, and dysarthria.
- Symptoms often fluctuate throughout the day and worsen with prolonged muscle use.
- There is usually no sensory, or cerebellar deficit nor abnormalities in the reflexes.
- Respiratory failure may be precipitated by infection, surgery, or rapid tapering of immunosuppressive medications.

Clinical Pearls

- Fluctuating diplopia, ptosis, slurred speech after prolonged periods of conversation, and food remaining in the mouth after swallowing are findings highly characteristic of MG (these findings often do not localize).
- The pupils are always normal in MG.
- Acute respiratory failure can occur from either acute myasthenic or cholineric crisis.
- Respiratory failure is a rare initial presentation of MG.
- 15–20 percent of MG patients will experience a myasthenic crisis during their lifetime.
- Common causes that precipitate a myasthenic crisis include infection, drug noncompliance or withdrawal, surgery and other physiological stressors; no cause is found in some patients.
- Some debate exists regarding rapid sequence intubation (RSI) for patients in myasthenic crisis, given concerns over prolonged paralysis and hyperkalemia.

- MG patients are extremely sensitive to both polarizing and nondepolarizing paralytic agents, and the effects of these medication may last more than three times as long as in normal patients. This is an important issue for anesthesiologists intubating a myasthenic patient for elective surgery.
- However, the average time a myasthenic crisis patient remains intubated is 13 days, making prolonged paralysis a far less important issue.
- Likewise, there is no upregulation of acetylcholine receptors; therefore, the risk of hyperkalemia is minimal.
- Suggested RSI modifications include using an induction agent without a paralytic (for severely weak patients) or using a smaller dose of a nondepolarizing agent (such as rocuronium).
- For all the aforementioned reasons, selecting the method that allows the best chance of initial success (usually standard RSI) makes the best sense.

Investigations

- Rest and acetylcholinesterase inhibitors transiently increase acetylcholine levels in the synaptic cleft and improve strength
- Cold temperature may also transiently improve strength. This is sometimes clinically useful at the bedside. In the evaluation of ptosis, improvement may be noted after several minutes of holding an ice pack to the affected eye in myasthenia. This is thought to be due either to reduced inactivation of acetylcholinesterase and/or prolonged opening of sodium channels.
- The diagnosis of MG may be established through the administration of edrophonium chloride (acetylcholinesterase inhibitor), electromyogram (EMG) studies, or serologic testing for AChR antibodies.
- Edrophonium increases the amount of acetylcholine at the neuromuscular junction.
- Edrophonium has a rapid onset (30 seconds) and a short duration of effect (5 to 10 minutes).
- In a myasthenic exacerbation, edrophonium should improve muscle weakness within a few minutes (Table 6.1).
- Caution should be used when administering edrophonium as it may cause bradycardia, atrioventricular block, atrial fibrillation, and cardiac arrest.
- Atropine will counteract the muscarinic effects, but not the nicotinic effects (skeletal muscle paralysis).
- EMG testing demonstrates a rapid reduction in muscle action potential with repetitive nerve stimulation.

119

Table 6.1 **Differentiation of Myasthenic vs. Cholinergic Crisis in Myasthenic Patients***

Characteristics	Myasthenic Crisis	Cholinergic Crisis
Etiology	Disease exacerbation (often precipitated by infection, surgery, medication noncompliance, or other physiological stressors) or inadequate drug therapy	Excessive cholinergic drug therapy resulting in excessive stimulation of acetylcholine receptors
Symptoms	Muscle weakness Respiratory failure	Muscle weakness Respiratory failure Muscarinic symptoms of sweating, salivation, lacrimation, miosis, tachycardia, gastrointestinal hyperactivity
Response to edrophonium	Improved muscle weakness	Muscle fasciculations, respiratory depression, or cholinergic symptoms (increased airway secretions, increased bowel motility)

*In some patients without a diagnosis of myasthenia, respiratory crisis can be the initial presentation.

Box 6.5 **The Tensilon (edrophonium) Test**

- Identify a visible target weak muscle to be tested.
- Prepare 2 mg of atropine to have available at bedside; ideally the patient should be on a cardiac monitor.
- Inject 1–2 mg of edrophonium intravenously over 15 seconds while observing improvement in target muscles.
- Improvement should occur within 30 seconds and disappear in 5 minutes.
- If no response and no significant adverse effects occur, administer an additional 8 mg (total dose of 10 mg).
- Atropine should be injected (0.5–1 mg) if clinically significant bradycardia, respiratory distress, or syncope occurs.

Edrophonium Dosing

Adult (IV): 1–2 mg (test dose) followed by up to 10 mg
Adult (IM): 10 mg

Children (IV): 0.2 mg/kg, not to exceed 10 mg
Children (IM): 2 mg

Box 6.6 The Ice Test

- Ice pack is applied to the more ptotic eye for 2 minutes.
- Improved ptosis indicates a positive test.
- A positive test strongly suggests a diagnosis of MG whereas a negative test decreases the likelihood.

- AChR antibody testing is the most specific test. However, up to 15 percent of MG patients may have undetectable antibody titers.

Management

- Cholinesterase inhibitors (pyridostigmine and neostigmine) are used for outpatient therapy.
- Immunosuppressive drugs such as corticosteroids, azathioprine, and cyclosporine have been used for chronic control of MG.
- Neurology consultation is recommended when using these agents.
- Thymectomy can be effective for those patients with thymoma.
- Plasma exchange and intravenous immunoglobulin (IVIg) are used for short-term immunomodulatory therapy in patients with severe exacerbations or during preoperative periods.
- Myasthenic crisis, defined as respiratory failure due to an exacerbation of myasthenia is a true neuromuscular emergency. The threshold for intubation should be low and is indicated in patients with clinical signs of respiratory distress (tachypnea, use of accessory muscles of respiration) or when simple bedside PFTs such as NIF and FVC are low or quickly trending downward. Some authorities recommend intubation if NIF is less than -15 or FVC is less than 15 cc/kg.
- In myasthenic crisis, be sure to treat the underlying cause.

Botulism

Food-borne botulism is caused by ingestion of a preformed toxin from Clostridium botulinum growing in improperly preserved or prepared foods. Canned foods are a common source, but other foods are not uncommon. In Alaska, whale and fish meat is a common source. However, because the spores are ubiquitous in nature, even foods such as vegetables and garlic packed in oil (which provides the anaerobic conditions) can lead to botulism. Infant botulism can occur after the ingestion of raw honey. Wound botulism most commonly occurs in intravenous drug users and in wounds grossly contaminated by the soil. Botulism toxin binds irreversibly to the presynaptic membrane at the neuromuscular junction preventing the release of acetylcholine from peripheral nerve synapses. The toxin blocks both voluntary and autonomic functions.

Presentation

- Symptoms occur within 24–48 hours.
- The most common symptoms include blurred vision, diplopia, and photophobia.
- Dysphagia, and dysarthria are also common.
- Trunk and extremity weakness often occurs in a symmetrical descending pattern.
- As the toxin blocks cholinergic output, anticholinergic signs may be present such as constipation, dry mouth, urinary retention, and fever.
- There are no sensory deficits and no pain.
- Respiratory failure is the most common cause of death and can occur within 6–8 hours of the onset of symptoms.
- Infantile symptoms include lethargy, poor feeding, a weak cry, and loss of head control.

Clinical Pearls

- Botulism spores are heat resistant; therefore, toxins may still be produced after thoroughly cooking foods. The toxin, however, is inactivated by heating foods to temperatures > 85 degrees C for 5 minutes (therefore, thoroughly heating foods prior to eating will prevent botulism.
- Mortality has decreased from 60 percent to 2–5 percent over the past 30 years.
- Acute cranial nerve dysfunction (ptosis, diplopia, dysarthria) is considered a hallmark of botulism.
- Botulism typically occurs in small clusters (2–3 cases), but sporadic cases also occur, in which case the diagnosis can be quite difficult.

Investigations

- Confirmation consists of demonstration of botulinum toxin in serum or stool or in food the patient has recently consumed.
- Electromyography (EMG) and nerve conduction studies (NCSs) may also demonstrate characteristic abnormalities, which may be helpful if the diagnosis is in question.
- Respiratory mechanics should be tested in the ED.

- If an LP is done because of concern for GBS or other problems, the CSF is normal.

Management

- Employ respiratory stabilization and supportive measures (endotracheal intubation if necessary).
- Antitoxin obtained from the state health department should be administered as soon as possible.
- Patients should be tested for hypersensitivity to horse serum prior to the administration.
- The CDC recommends that clinicians contact their state health department with suspected cases.
- Updated information can be found on the CDC Emergency Preparedness and Response web site:
  - http://emergency.cdc.gov/agent/botulism
- CDC Emergency Operations Center (for healthcare professionals):
  - (770) 488-7100

Tick Paralysis

Tick paralysis is caused by a tick-injected toxin that decreases the release of acetylcholine at the neuromuscular junction and reduces the velocity of nerve conduction. More than 60 species of ticks have been associated with paralysis.

Presentation

- Acute, ascending symmetrical paralysis that evolves over hours to days.
- Symptoms usually begin 1 to 5 days following the tick exposure.
- Ocular signs may occur, such a fixed and dilated pupils.
- DTRs are diminished or absent.
- Respiratory paralysis and death can occur.
- Prodromal symptoms of paresthesias, restlessness, irritability, fatigue, and myalgias may be present.
- Children may be more susceptible to the paralytic agent given their lower body weight.
- Young girls, probably because of difficulty finding ticks in long hair, seem to be inordinately affected.

Clinical Pearls

- Fever is absent.
- Tick paralysis mimics GBS and, therefore, all patients with suspected GBS should be carefully examined for ticks.
- Examination should focus on the scalp, axilla, and groin— areas that may escape detection with a superficial examination.

- Symptoms occasionally persist or even worsen after removal of the tick.
- Patients may have more than one tick attached.

Investigations

- Ticks are most commonly found in the scalp, behind the ear, or in the groin, axilla, or perineum.
- If tested, CSF, CT, and MRI studies are normal; none of these tests is necessary if a tick is found.

Management

- Supportive and respiratory care is needed.
- Definitive therapy is removal of the tick.
- Symptoms usually improve within hours of tick removal.

Myopathies

Periodic Paralysis

Periodic paralysis may occur as a result of numerous clinical syndromes, many related to inherited genetic mutations, causing dysfunction of voltage-sensitive membrane channels. Two of the most common causes of periodic paralysis are hypokalemic paralysis and hyperkalemic paralysis.

Hypokalemic periodic paralysis (HPP) can be subdivided into familial periodic paralysis (FPP) or thyrotoxic periodic paralysis (TPP). FPP is an autosomal dominant disorder associated with a mutation involving voltage-gated calcium channel. TPP is similar and often clinically indistinguishable to hypokalemic FPP, but associated with hyperthyroidism. Hyperthyroidism is a hyperadrenergic state that causes B2-adrenergic stimulation in muscle cells directly inducing cellular potassium uptake. Attacks of weakness are relatively infrequent but severe.

Hyperkalemic periodic paralysis is inherited in an autosomal dominant pattern and is due to one of several changes in the skeletal muscle sodium channel gene, SCN4A. Patients may develop myotonia due to a small depolarization and repetitive excitation; however, more commonly develop paralysis due to inexcitability. Attacks of weakness are typically frequent but not as severe as in hypokalemic periodic paralysis.

Presentation

- Periodic paralysis is characterized by recurrent episodes of flaccid paralysis.
- Onset is usually rapid and may last 6 to 24 hours.
- It is more common in males and Asian patients.

- Initial attacks often occur in teenage years.
- Mental status and sensation are usually unaffected.
- The lower extremities are more often involved than upper extremities.
- Bulbar, ocular, and respiratory muscles are usually not involved.
- TPP may present with hypertension and tachycardia, however some patients do not have symptoms related to hyperthyroidism.
- Tachycardia may be present in cases associated with hyperthyroidism.
- A goiter may be present in thyrotoxic patients.
- An irregular pulse is common secondary to PVCs due to hypokalemia.

Clinical Pearls

- Patients will often report a history (or family history) of similar occurrences.
- Attacks of hypokalemic paralysis may be induced by excess carbohydrate intake or injection of glucose, insulin, or epinephrine (increase cellular potassium uptake).
- Hyperkalemic paralysis may occur after periods of strenuous exercise or after ingesting foods rich in potassium such as fruits.
- Beta-blocking agents should be avoided in hyperkalemia as they can impede cellular potassium uptake.
- Likewise, depolarizing anesthetic agents should be avoided as they can evoke potassium release from cells and also place patients at risk for malignant hyperthermia.
- In addition to the disorders discussed previously, it is worth noting that profound hyper or hypokalemia (due to an underlying medical illness) as well as hypermagnesemia or hypophosphatemia may also lead to acute flaccid weakness.

Investigations

- ECG may demonstrate signs of hypokalemia or hyperkalemia.
- An immediate potassium level should be obtained.
- Hypokalemic forms of paralysis often have value below 3.0 mEq/L.
- Patients with HPP should be evaluated for thyrotoxicosis.
- The occurrence of paralysis in conjunction with an abnormal potassium level and a family history of the disorder are diagnostic.
- Genetic testing can also confirm the diagnosis.

Management

- Most cases resolve with supportive care and correction of serum potassium levels.
- Treatment of hypokalemia:
  - 10–20 mEq of potassium over one hour

- 40 mEq orally
- Treatment of hyperkalemia:
  - Calcium gluconate (minimizes membrane excitability)
  - Glucose/Insulin (stimulates cellular potassium uptake)
  - Beta2-agonists (also stimulates cellular uptake)
  - Kayexalate (binds and removes potassium from the body)

Box 6.7 Caution Regarding Treatment of Hypokalemic Paralysis

Because total body stores of potassium are normal in this condition, caution should be used when treating hypokalemia because over treatment can lead to hyperkalemia. Retesting of potassium levels is recommended.

Spinal Cord Disorders

Transverse Myelitis

Transverse myelitis is characterized by acute or subacute paraplegia, a distinct transverse level of sensory impairment, and autonomic disturbances. Autonomic symptoms may include urinary urgency, bowel or bladder incontinence, incomplete evacuation, and constipation. Transverse myelitis is caused by a spinal cord dysfunction that may be infectious, toxic, autoimmune, or idiopathic in origin. It is most commonly due to a postviral or toxic inflammation of the spinal cord (including radiation effects during cancer therapy). No apparent cause for acute transverse myelitis is found in up to 30 percent of patients.

Presentation

- The clinical course is variable.
- Symptoms often rapidly progress (maximal within 24 hours).
- Numbness, paresthias, and band-like dysesthesias are very common. Patients may describe their sensory symptoms as a pressure or band-like" sensation (e.g., like a tight waist band or bra strap). Other descriptors include the sensation of the skin feeling like wax paper or that their limbs feel thick or swollen.
- Approximately 50 percent of patients will lose all movement of their legs when the maximal level of deficit is reached.
- The thoracic cord is most often affected.
- Virtually all patients have bladder dysfunction.
- Maximal improvement usually occurs within 3–6 months.
- Approximately one-third are left with moderate disability, one-third with severe disability, and one-third recover with little or no sequelae.

Clinical Pearls

- The presentation may mimic a compressive lesion, spinal cord infarction, or trauma.
- Testing of posterior column functions (vibration, proprioception) is critical, because these are often affected in patients with transverse myelitis and spared in those with a cord infarct due to occlusion of the anterior spinal artery or one of its parent vessels (discussed later).
- Testing for a sensory level with pin is also critically important. Though a sensory level may be indicative of the level of the pathology in the cord, it is not always the case. Once a sensory level is determined, it is crucial to continue to assess more rostral levels, because "skip areas" with sensory sparing are well described. In other words, once a sensory level is found on exam, the lesion is typically at that level or higher. This may have implications in determining which levels of the spinal cord (cervical or thoracic) to image.
- Transverse myelitis may be either complete (involving the entire cord) or incomplete (only involving a portion of the transverse area of the cord). In these latter cases, the examination may be patchy or asymmetric, leading to diagnostic confusion. In these instances, other processes need to be ruled out (particularly spinal cord compression and metastases).
- Symptoms follow a viral infection in approximately 30 percent of patents.
- Transverse myelitis can be the presenting feature of multiple sclerosis and Lyme disease.

Investigations

MRI and lumber puncture often show evidence of acute inflammation (see Figure 6.2)

- MRI is also crucial to rule out other causes of spinal cord pathology (particularly those requiring immediate medical and surgical treatment), such as cord compression (either due to neoplastic disease; infection, such as an epidural abscess; or hematoma) and infarction.
- Inflammation within the spinal cord is demonstrated by CSF pleocytosis.

Management

- Steroids are controversial as some studies have found no benefit to their use.
- Admission and neurology consultation is recommended.
- Other rare causes of spinal cord dysfunction, such as tuberculosis, schistosomiasis, Lyme disease, syphilis, and varicella zoster virus infection should be considered if risk factors are present, because

CHAPTER 6 Generalized Weakness

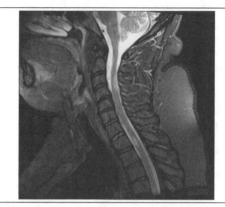

Figure 6.2 Transverse Myelitis. A STIR MRI image demonstrates a partial transverse myelitis at two levels (C3 and T1) in a 43-year-old patient with multiple sclerosis.

Table 6.2 **Comparative Characteristics**				
	GBS	**Botulism**	**Tick Paralysis**	**Transverse myelitis**
Fever	Rare	Absent	Absent	Variable
Pain	Rare	Absent	Rare	Frequent
Sensory findings	Often	Absent	Rare	Frequent
Dilated pupils	Rare	Present	Rare	Absent
CSF protein	Elevated	Normal	Normal	Often elevated
CSF wbc	Normal	Normal	Normal	Elevated
MRI	Normal	Normal	Normal	Abnormal

specific antibiotic treatment is warranted in these cases.

Table 6.2 summarizes some of the features that distinguishes transverse myelitis from GBS, Botulism, and Tick paralysis.

Spinal Cord Compression

Spinal cord compression is a true neurologic emergency. Early diagnosis and treatment are essential to ensure a successful long-term functional outcome. The major causes of spinal cord compression are neoplastic, non-neoplastic, and traumatic. Neoplastic and non-neoplastic causes typically lead to subacute and at times insidious onset of symptoms, whereas traumatic causes produce acute symptoms.

Presentation

- Most patients will complain of axial spine pain. This is typically worse at night and when supine in patients with neoplastic causes of compression.
- Patients with nerve root involvement may also complain of radicular symptoms.
- On examination, pain to palpation or percussion over a particular region of the spine may be indicative of the level involved.
- Examination typically demonstrates signs of spinal shock below the level of the lesion, including flaccid paralysis, lack of sensation to all modalities, and absent reflexes. Evaluation for a spinal sensory level is critical and may indicate the level of the lesion. In addition, urinary retention is common.
- In patients with spinal epidural abscess the presenting symptoms involve a triad of back pain, fever, and spinal shock below the level of the lesion. Unfortunately, only a minority of patients have the full triad at initial presentation. Fever is only present in half of cases.
- Also, in spinal epidural abscess, leukocytosis is only present in two-thirds of cases, although the inflammatory markers, such as elevated ESR or CRP, are usually elevated.

Clinical Pearls

- The most common neoplastic cause for spinal cord compression is from metastases. Frequent tumors causing cord compression include those arising from breast, lung, prostate, kidney, as well as from multiple myeloma and lymphoma. Primary spinal cord tumors are much less common.
- The thoracic cord is most frequently affected in neoplastic cord compression.
- Cervical spondylotic arthropathy is the most common non-neoplastic cause of cord compression and typically evolves insidiously; however, acute traumatic disc herniation can cause cord compression that presents acutely.
- Spinal epidural abscess is a more serious cause of non-neoplastic cord compression. Risk factors for the development of spinal epidural abscess include immunocompromised state, diabetes mellitus, intravenous drug use, chronic kidney disease, and/or a history of spinal injury or surgery.
- The most common organisms involved in spinal epidural abscesses are Staphylococcus aureus, coagulase-negative Staphylococcus, and Gram negative organisms. Tuberculosis is another common cause in underdeveloped nations.
- Spinal epidural abscesses are frequently associated with concomitant discitis and/or osteomyelitis.

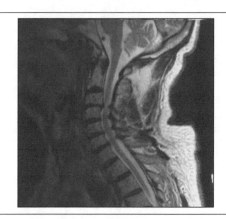

Figure 6.3 Cord Compression. A T2 weighted MRI image of cervical spinal cord compression in an 83-year-old patient with severe cervical spondyolosis. Note the multi-level degenerative bony changes impinging on both the ventral and dorsal aspects of the cord.

Investigations

- Regardless of the cause, any patient suspected of suffering from spinal cord compression should undergo an emergent MRI of the entire spine (with sagittal and coronal reformats) with and without gadolinium. MRI is preferred as it is more able to evaluate both nonosseous as well as osseous structures (see Figure 6.3).

- If a patient is unable to undergo MRI due to the presence of a pacemaker, significant claustrophobia, or other contraindications, CT myelography is an acceptable alternative, though it is more invasive and requires staff experienced in performing this procedure.

- In patients with spinal epidural abscess, lumbar puncture is contraindicated due to the risk of puncturing the abscess and causing further spread of organisms. CSF cultures are rarely positive in patients with this condition, whereas blood cultures drawn before the institution of antibiotic therapy often identify the causative organism.

Management

- In patients with neoplastic cord compression, immediate treatment with intravenous dexamethasone (10 mg) is warranted, followed by 4 mg IV every six hours.

- Emergent consultation with a spine surgeon is also warranted because early decompression and stabilization have been shown to be of most benefit in the first 24 to 48 hours after the development of symptoms.

- In patients with radiosensitive tumors (particularly lymphoma and myeloma), emergent radiation therapy is also employed in most cases.
- In patients with spinal epidural abscesses, treatment consists of intravenous antibiotics and surgical decompression/debridement of the abscess.

Box 6.8 Spinal Cord Trauma

Spinal cord dysfunction is the most common cause of severe disability after trauma. It is standard of care to assume that every trauma patient has suffered an injury to the cord and be immobilized until spinal injuries are ruled out. A search for concomitant injuries must be performed in patients with spinal injury because other injuries are common in this population. Treatment with steroids in the acute phase is controversial and has, at best, a modest effect on outcome but may result in more frequent complications (particularly pulmonary infections).

Spinal Cord Infarction

Spinal cord infarction is much more rare than brain infarction. A high index of suspicion is often required to make the diagnosis. The vascular supply of the spinal cord consists of one single anterior spinal artery and two paired posterior spinal arteries. The anterior spinal artery nourishes the anterior two-thirds of the cord in a transverse plane, whereas the posterior spinal arteries supply the posterior third, which predominantly consists of the dorsal columns. The anterior spinal artery is formed from contributions of both vertebral arteries, which descend through the foramen magnum to reach the cord. There are several (5–10) radicular arteries that subsequently feed the anterior spinal artery as it descends, the largest of which typically arises in the T9 to T12 region and is referred to as the artery of Adamkiewicz. The blood supply to the anterior spinal cord is most marginal in the lower thoracic and upper lumbar cord, and spinal cord infarcts most frequently occur at these levels. Unlike the anterior spinal artery, the posterior spinal arteries receive collateral flow from radicular arteries at just about every level, and, therefore, infarcts in their territory are much less frequent.

Presentation

- Spinal cord infarcts are often precipitated by exertion.
- Pain in the neck or back commonly precedes other symptoms by minutes to hours.

- Overwhelmingly, infarcts involve the anterior portion of the cord (supplied by the anterior spinal artery) and patients present with flaccid paralysis and loss of pain and temperature sensation below the level of the infarct, with sparing of dorsal column functions of proprioception and vibratory sensation.
- Although most often bilateral, infarcts in the distribution of the anterior spinal artery may be unilateral and present with a Brown-Sequard syndrome (weakness on the side of the infarct, with loss of pain and temperature on the contralateral side below the level of the lesion).

Clinical Pearls

- The cause of spinal cord infarcts is not found in most cases.
- Known causes include disease of the aorta (including rupture aneurysm, dissection, or as a complication of aortic surgery). Thromboembolic occlusion (for example in endocarditis or from embolization of intravertebral discs), heroin or cocaine use, or venous infarction due to underlying spinal-dural arteriovenous malformations or coagulopathies are other recognized causes.
- Systemic hypotension is another cause of spinal cord infarction, though typically concomitant infarction of the brain overshadows the diagnosis.
- Spinal cord hemorrhages are even more rare than infarction and are most often due to trauma, coagulopathies, use of anticoagulation, or underlying arteriovenous malformations.

Investigations

- MRI with diffusion-weighted imaging is the diagnostic imaging modality of choice.
- Typically, infarction is best visualized on sagittal images.

Management

- There is no specific treatment other than prevention of further episodes of infarction, and care is largely supportive.
- There have been no studies of anticoagulation or antithrombotic therapy. However, some studies have shown modest benefit with placement of lumbar drains to relieve spinal pressure.
- Patients should be admitted for evaluation, stabilization, and institution of physical therapy.

Suggested Readings

Benatar M. Neurological potassium channelopathies. *QJM*. 2000;93:787–797.

Bleecker JL, et al. Neurological manifestations of organophosphate poisoning. *Clin Neurol Neurosurg*. 1992;94:93–103.

Bracken MB, Shepard MJ, Collins WF, et al. A randomized, controlled trial of methylprednisolone or naloxone in the treatment of acute spinal-cord injury. Results of the Second National Acute Spinal Cord Injury Study. *N Engl J Med.* 1990;322:1405–1411.

Darouiche RLO. Spinal epidural abscess. *NEJM.* 2006;355:2012–2020.

Edlow JA, McGillicuddy DC. Tick paralysis. *Infect Dis Clin N Am.* 2008;22:397–413.

Scherer K, Bedlack RS, Simel DL. Does this patient have Myasthenia Gravis? *JAMA.* 2005;293:1906–1914.

Shapiro RL, Hatheway C, Swerdlow DL. Botulism in the United States: a clinical and epidemiologic review. *Ann Intern Med.* 1998;129:221–228.

Transverse Myelitis Consortium Working Group. Proposed diagnostic criteria and nosology of acute transverse myelitis. *Neurology.* 2002;59:499–505.

VanDoorn PA, Ruts L, Jacobs BC. Clinical features, pathogenesis, and treatment of Guillain-Barre syndrome. *Lancet Neurol.* 2008;7:939–950.

Winters ME, Kluetz P, Zilberstein J. Back pain emergencies. *Med Clin North Am.* 2006;90:505–523.

Chapter 7

CNS Infections

J. Stephen Huff and Barnett R. Nathan

Introduction

Central nervous system (CNS) infections cover the spectrum of clinical acuity from rapidly progressive bacterial infections to slow and even indolent infections by viral and prion agents. The CNS is an immunologically privileged site. Host-infectious agent interactions determine the tempo of the infectious process, as do individual anatomic variations. The diagnostic strategy may be straightforward or circuitous. As with other clinical conditions, the work-up at the initial patient encounter is driven by the pretest probability that a CNS infection is present. The clinician is still dependent on a thorough history and physical examination to set clinical likelihoods and direct further work-up. Additional diagnostic tools include neuroimaging studies and lumbar puncture.

Acute bacterial meningitis remains a significant cause of morbidity and mortality throughout the world and receives emphasis. Age-based treatment regimens for meningitis are presented as well as diagnostic strategies. Other syndromes that are bacterial in origin, but that assume specific clinical syndromes, such as cerebral subdural abscess and spinal epidural abscess, are also delineated.

The immunosuppressed patient warrants special considerations. The patient with HIV infection, whether a new diagnosis or with medically refractory disease, increases the risk of CNS infection from toxoplasmosis, tuberculosis, Cryptococcus, and other agents. A wider differential diagnosis must be cast in this patient population.

Bacterial Meningitis

Pathophysiology

- Most bacteria causing meningitis gain access to the central nervous system by hematogenous spread from distant sites of infection. Sources include respiratory tract infections, endocarditis, distant abscesses, catheters, shunts, and implanted medical devices.
- Bacteremia and a breach of the blood-brain barrier allow entry of the organism into the CNS.
- Direct extension from sinus or ear infections may occur.
- Inflammatory responses with neuronal injury follow.
- Vasculitis and cerebral edema may occur.
- Bacterial agents that commonly affect patients are often age-related.
  - Age < 30 days—Group B strep, *E. Coli*, Listeria, Klebsiella.

- Children and adults—Neisseria meningitidis, H. influenza, S. pneumoniae.
- Adults > 50 years—Neisseria meningitidis, S. pneumoniae, Listeria, Gram negatives.
- Penetrating injuries and postsurgical infections have a different profile of infectious agents including *S. aureus* and *S. epidermidis*.

History and Physical Examination

- In infants, poor feeding and irritability may be the presenting symptoms.
- History may include elements of confusion, fever, seizure, or headache.
- Diabetes and alcoholism are often cited as predisposing factors.
- Cerebral functioning and mental status generally remain intact or are only mildly impaired.
- Fever on presentation is the rule, but occasional patients may be afebrile.
- Nuchal rigidity may be a valuable clue if present, but the absence of neck stiffness does not exclude meningitis.
- The jolt accentuation of headache maneuver is more valuable for evaluating meningeal irritation than Kernig's or Brudzinski's maneuvers.
  - The jolt accentuation of headache maneuver is elicited by asking the patient to turn their head horizontally at 2–3 rotations per second (as if the patient were shaking their head to indicate "no"). Ask if the headache worsens.
  - A positive test is the patient grimacing or responding that the headache worsens.
- A rash may be present in meningococcal or (less commonly) with pneumococcal infections.

Clinical Pearls

- Once a suspicion of bacterial meningitis is present, antibiotic therapy and adjunctive therapy should not be delayed pending neuroimaging or lumbar puncture.
- Peripheral blood cultures are often positive in cases of bacterial meningitis and should be obtained.
- Adjunctive use of dexamethasone in adults is recommended at or before the time of antibiotic administration. Dexamethasone use is beneficial in studies involving patients with proven meningitis, mostly with pneumococcal meningitis. Risk and benefits of steroid use in the larger patient population with suspected meningitis that receive antibiotics before CSF is examined has not been thoroughly studied.

- Seizures may occur as part of the meningitis syndrome.
- Tuberculous meningitis, technically a bacterial meningitis, may present with a CSF formula with lymphocytic predominance. Patients appear ill, and additional clinical features, such as immunosuppression or immigration from an endemic area, are often present.

Investigations

- Cranial noncontrast CT scan is commonly performed before lumbar puncture to evaluate for mass effect or signs of increased intracranial pressure.
- Lumbar puncture may be performed without cranial CT in patients in whom physical examination shows no focal abnormalities, no papilledema, and normal level of consciousness.
  - In bacterial meningitis, the CSF white blood cell count will be elevated, most often with segmented form predominance (Table 7.1).
  - Glucose is reduced.
  - Protein will be elevated.
  - If obtained, lactic acid may be elevated.
  - Opening pressure may be elevated.
  - CSF may be visibly cloudy.
  - Subtle cloudiness may be quickly established by attempting to read print viewing through a tube of CSF.

Management

- Prompt recognition and intervention in patients with acute bacterial meningitis is the goal of emergency care.
- Airway management and circulatory support may be necessary in some patients.
- Therapy should be initiated promptly when suspicion for bacterial meningitis reasonably enters the differential diagnosis.

Table 7.1 CSF Formula for Differentiation of Bacterial and Nonbacterial Meningitis

	Normal	Bacterial meningitis	Nonbacterial meningitis
WBC count	< 5	Elevated, often > 1,000	<1,000
Cell types		> 80% PMN	< 20% PMN
Glucose	45–60	Reduced	Normal or minimally reduced
Protein	20–45	High	High (usually less so than with bacterial)

Table 7.2 **Age-related common bacterial causes of meningitis and recommended medications**

Age	Common Organisms	Recommended Medications Pending Identification
Neonate	*Listeria* Gram negatives Group B Strep	Third generation cephalosporin Ampicillin
Children and adults < 50 years	Pneumococcus Meningococcus *H. Influenza*	Third generation cephalosporin Vancomycin
Adults > 50 years	Pneumococcus Gram negatives Listeria	Third generation cephalosporin Vancomycin Ampicillin

- Initial antibiotic therapy is empiric, age-based to correspond with likely organisms, and involves multiple drugs (Table 7.2).
  - Age < 30 days—ampicillin, ceftriaxone
  - Children and adults—third generation cephalosporin (e.g., ceftriaxone), vancomycin
  - Adults > 50 years—third generation cephalosporin (e.g., ceftriaxone), vancomycin, ampicillin
  - Hospital-acquired—vancomycin and antipseudomonal cephalosporin
- Steroids should be given at the time of antibiotics or moments before in cases of acute bacterial meningitis in adults.
  - Reductions in adverse outcomes and death is especially important in the occasional patient with Waterhouse-Friderichsen syndrome (circulatory collapse from adrenal hemorrhage in the setting of disseminated meningococcal disease).
  - Adults—Dexamethasone 0.15 mg/kg q6 hours for 2–4 days with the first dose administered 10–20 minutes before or concomitant with the first dose of antimicrobial therapy.
  - Pediatrics—If used, dexamethasone as above (studies are conflicting regarding efficacy).
- Chemoprophylaxis should be offered household contacts and healthcare providers with secretion exposures in cases of *Neisseria meningitides*.
  - Rifampin, ciprofloxacin, ceftriaxone, and azithromycin are among the recommended agents, with ciprofloxacin now the preferred agent in adults due to its ease of dosing (single 500 mg oral dose) and the relative lack of adverse reactions.

- An immunosuppressed host should prompt consideration of other agents such as tuberculosis and nonbacterial agents, such as toxoplasmosis and Cryptococcus.
- Tuberculous meningitis cases will need multiple antibiotic coverage.
  - Four-drug treatment is initially recommended, which may include isoniazid, rifampin, pyrazinamide, streptomycin, or ethambutol.
  - Treatment for months is often needed.
  - Adjunctive steroid use is recommended.
  - Consultation with infectious disease recommended.

Nonbacterial Meningitis

The grouping of several different infectious agents under the title of nonbacterial meningitis serves to distinguish these presentations from that of acute bacterial meningitis. Often *aseptic meningitis* is used almost synonymously with meningitis of viral etiology, but the term is perhaps best discarded. *Aseptic meningitis* refers to the lack of bacterial growth in CSF cultures and is a misnomer because most cases are caused by various viruses, and Lyme or tuberculous meningitis are bacterial causes. The clinical presentation will be that of headache and perhaps altered mental status. However, this may be misleading, because within this grouping the clinical course may range from mild headache to a progressive syndrome of altered mental status with significant morbidity and mortality if untreated. Treatments vary depending on the etiologic organism. CSF analysis generally shows a lymphocytic predominance, and a white count lower than that of acute bacterial meningitis.

Pathophysiology

- Entry into the CSF is often from respiratory route with hematogenous seeding in most cases.
- Seeding from other sites may take place as well.
- Enteroviruses and Herpes Simplex Virus (HSV) are common causes of adult nonbacterial meningitis.
- Many others may produce a similar clinical picture.

History and Physical Examination

- History is usually nonspecific with complaints of headache and general malaise.
- Fever may or may not be present.
- Physical examination may show signs of meningeal irritation.
- Mental status alteration is mild.

Clinical Pearls

- Chronic steroid therapy is a risk factor for cryptococcal infections.
- Although enteroviruses tend to produce meningitic syndromes, and arboviruses tend to produce encephalitic syndromes, exceptions do occur.
- HIV-associated cryptococcal infection accounts for 80–90 percent of cases of cryptococcal meningitis and in many patients is the AIDS-defining illness.

Investigations

- For patients with altered mental status, neuroimaging, such as cranial CT, is usually initiated on presentation to the emergency department.
- For patients with a more indolent course, MRI may have been obtained and may show evidence of meningeal involvement.
- Lumbar puncture often shows a nonspecific lymphocytic predominance of white blood cells, with modestly depressed glucose and modestly increased protein.
- Bacteria are absent on Gram's strain.
- India ink testing may be useful in cases of suspected cryptococcal meningitis to reveal the organism.
- Cryptococcal antigen assay of CSF may be positive in some cases when India ink testing is negative.
- Specific antigenic testing may be available for select viruses.
- Etiology often remains unclear even following extensive testing.
- If Lyme disease is considered, serological testing of the blood and/or the CSF are recommended.

Management

- Following CSF analysis, therapy can be tailored if a specific infectious agent is discovered.
- If bacterial meningitis is reasonably in the differential diagnosis, appropriate antibacterial therapy should be continued until cultures or other laboratory testing excludes that as a diagnostic possibility (see preceding section)
- If HSV is reasonably in the differential diagnosis, acyclovir should be initiated and continued until that diagnosis is excluded (see section that follow).
- Varicella zoster viral infections may cause a picture of meningoencephalitis and are also responsive to acyclovir.
- Fungal meningitis from *Cryptococcus neoformans* should be treated with amphotericin 0.7 mg/kg/d in combination with flucytosine 200 mg/kg/d.

• Lyme meningitis is typically treated with IV ceftriaxone although some studies suggest that PO doxycycline may be adequate.

Encephalitis

Pathophysiology

• When infectious or inflammatory processes present with cortical findings, such as aphasia, personality changes, hemiparesis or other focal findings, cortical involvement is implied, and the process is referred to as an encephalitis.

• Encephalitis and meningitis exist on a continuum; meningoencephalitis often more accurately describes the observed pathology.

• Many types of encephalitis are of viral etiology, and a vector, often a mosquito, plays a role.

• Seasonal variation is present with arboviral infections, and is related to the prevalence of the vector.

• HSV encephalitis occurs sporadically, and most often follows reactivation of virus in the trigeminal ganglia.

• Disseminated HSV-1 disease may occur in neonates or in the immunosuppressed patient.

• Rabies and other uncommon viral infections fall under this diagnostic umbrella but are outside the scope of this chapter

History and Physical Examination

• History may give a clue of cerebral involvement, such as personality change.

• Fever is often present.

• Meningismus may be present.

• Physical examination may suggest a focal abnormality of the central nervous system such as aphasia or hemiparesis.

• Tremors, other movement disorders, or flaccid paralysis may occur with West Nile encephalitis.

Clinical Pearls

• HSV encephalitis is the most common sporadically occurring viral encephalitis with specific treatment.

• Encephalitis should be treated empirically as herpes simplex encephalitis pending culture or other laboratory results.

• HSV virus has a predilection for the temporal lobes, and imaging may show temporal lobe abnormalities (Figure 7.1).

• Seizures may occur with meningitis or encephalitis.

• Though there are many different viral types of encephalitis including St. Louis encephalitis, California virus, eastern equine

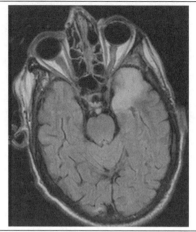

Figure 7.1 MRI of patient with Herpes Simplex encephalitis showing temporal lobe abnormality.

encephalitis, western equine encephalitis, West Nile virus, rabies, and others, only HSV encephalitis and Varicella encephalitis have specific treatment.

- CNS toxoplasmosis will often show many small lesions imaging and is rare unless the patient is immunosuppressed.

Investigations

- Neuroimaging should be performed in patients with altered mental status or neurologic deficits on examination.
- CSF will usually show an elevated WBC count (but less high than with acute bacterial meningitis).
- Lymphocytic predominance is often present in the CSF.
- Glucose and protein measurements of the CSF will be normal or only minimally abnormal.
- Polymerase chain reaction (PCR), testing for viral nucleic acids, is the current diagnostic test is available for HSV, and some arboviruses.
- CNS toxoplasmosis is usually discovered with characteristic multiple lesions on neuroimaging.

Management

- Pending definitive viral identification with PCR, acyclovir (Zovirax) is often initiated in the ill patient with herpes simplex virus in the differential diagnosis.

- Initial dose of acyclovir is 10–15 mg/kg, to be repeated every 8 hours.
- Arbovirus and enterovirus infections do not respond to acyclovir and the only treatment is supportive.
- If seizures occur they should be treated in the usual manner with benzodiazepines and a phenytoin.

Brain Abscess

Pathophysiology

- Most bacterial organisms gain access to the central nervous system by hematogenous spread.
- Direct extension may occur from dental, otogenic, and sinus sources.
- A penetrating injury with inoculation of the brain is another path of entry.
- Cardiac disease with right to left shunting and chronic lung disease have historically been risk factors for brain abscess.
- Brain abscess from intrapulmonary right to left shunting is an important cause of morbidity and mortality in patients with hereditary hemorrhagic telangectasia (HHT, or Osler-Weber-Rendu syndrome).

History and Physical Examination

- Often brain abscess presents a mass lesion with headaches or focal neurologic findings; the specific findings are a function on the area of the brain involved.
- A febrile meningitis-like presentation may occur.

Clinical Pearls

- Metastatic lesions are in the differential diagnosis of any patient with multiple intracranial lesions.
- Multiple lesions suggest the possibility of an immunosuppressed host and toxoplasmosis.
- A history of recurrent epistaxis or a family history of brain abscess suggests the possibility of HHT.
- Many patients with brain abscess will not have fever or leukocytosis.

Investigations

- Cranial computed tomography will usually demonstrate mass effect, edema, and midline shift; use of IV contrast will often show "ring enhancement" around the abscess (Figures 7.2 and 7.3).

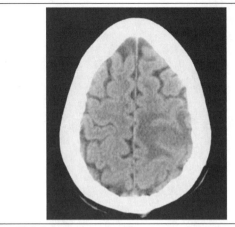

Figure 7.2 Brain abscess noncontrast CT.

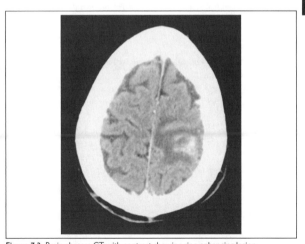

Figure 7.3 Brain abscess CT with contrast showing ring-enhancing lesion.

- When available, MRI has become the preferred imaging choice because it shows much greater detail than does CT (Figure 7.3).
- Lumbar puncture is usually contraindicated. Besides the issue of potential brain herniation, the CSF is very low yield in terms of identifying the causative organism.

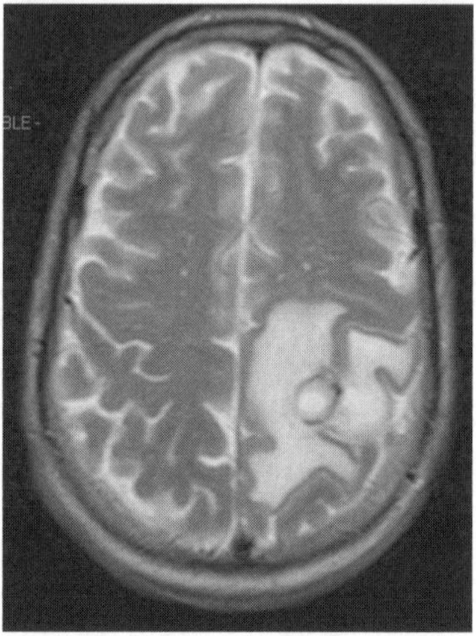

Figure 7.4 MRI of brain abscess showing surrounding edema and contrast enhancing ring.

Management

- Steroids (dexamethasone) may be useful in the patient with edema or mass effect.
- For the stable patient, antibiotic therapy may be deferred until neurosurgical aspiration of the abscess identifies a specific organism.
- For febrile or toxic patients, empiric antibiotic administration is indicated. Typically, coverage is with broad spectrum covering Gram positives (including MRSA), Gram negatives, and anaerobes. Antipseudomonals are rarely needed empirically unless the patient has risk factors for acquiring *Pseudomonas*.

Subdural Empyema

Pathophysiology

- Subdural infection involves the anatomic space between the dura and neural tissue.
- 95 percent of subdural infections are located intracranially
- Inflammatory process may extend over the brain and penetrate the parenchyma, causing cerebral edema and mass effect.
- Frequently, the empyema is an extension of a purulent sinusitis, and subdural empyema is most commonly present over the frontal lobes.

- Subdural empyema rarely may be present in the spinal subdural space, with back pain and radiculopathy being the presenting symptoms.

History and Physical Examination

- History of recent sinusitis or otitis media is often present.
- Headache may be unilateral or generalized.
- Fever and vomiting may be present.
- Focal or generalized seizures may occur.
- Most patients have altered mental status
- Focal neurologic signs such as hemiparesis or aphasia may be present.
- The tempo of the illness is often one of rapid progression.

Clinical Pearls

- Most cases are extensions of paranasal sinus infections.
- Subdural empyema may be a rapidly progressive process if untreated and has a significant mortality.

Investigations

- Cranial noncontrast CT scan is the rapid imaging study of choice.
- A subdural fluid collection in the appropriate clinical setting suggests the diagnosis.
- Lumbar puncture is contraindicated (and low yield).

Management

- Airway management and circulatory support may be necessary in some cases.
- Surgical evacuation of the empyema is the treatment of choice.
- Antibiotic therapy should be initiated toward *Staph aureus*, the most common pathogen.
- If a neurosurgical procedure has recently been performed, additional antibiotic coverage may be indicated.

Spinal Epidural Abscess

Pathophysiology

- Epidural infection involves the anatomic space between bone and the dura.
- In the spine, this space is filled with epidural fat, a venous plexus, and small arteries.
- Because of the anatomic constructs, over 90 percent of epidural infections occur along the spinal neuraxis.

- Most spinal epidural abscesses occur posteriorly, where the posterior epidural is large.
- Spinal epidural abscesses often spread over several vertebral levels.
- Hematogenous spread to the epidural space is the most common mechanism of abscess formation, with sources including urinary tract infections, indwelling catheters, endocarditis, abdominal abscesses, and others.
- Epidural injections and epidural catheters may be iatrogenic causes, as well as spinal surgery and lumbar puncture.
- Spinal cord involvement can be a result of either direct compression or impairment of the vascular supply to the cord.
- Common organisms include *Staph aureus*, but many different organisms have caused abscesses including Gram-negative rods, *Streptococcus* spp., *Enterococcus* spp., and others.

History and Physical Examination

- Early presentations may be subtle and indistinguishable from musculoskeletal low back pain.
- History of fever is often but not invariably present.
- Intravenous drug abuse, alcoholism, diabetes, and immunosuppression are predisposing conditions.
- Duration of symptoms may be abrupt or the symptoms may evolve over a few days or weeks.
- Radicular pain may be present and confound diagnosis, particularly if the pain is in abdominal or thoracic regions.
- Signs of spinal cord injury may be present with sphincter dysfunction.
- Transverse spinal cord syndrome is the most common spinal cord syndrome with paraplegia and sensory levels.
- Anterior cord syndrome and Brown-Sequard partial cord syndromes have also been reported.
- Reflexes may vary from hyperactive to absent, and pathologic reflexes may or may not be present.

Clinical Pearls

- High index of suspicion is the key to early diagnosis with particular attention to the patient with predisposing factors.
- Fever and leukocytosis may be absent.
- Erythrocyte sedimentation rate is usually elevated and may be useful as a screening tool in patients with low pretest probability of spinal epidural abscess.
- Some patients will have a slow progression of symptoms followed by an abrupt loss of neurological function due to a vascular infarct from a septic phlebitis or arteritis of the cord.

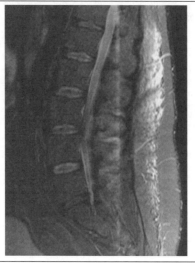

Figure 7.5 Spinal epidural abscess showing inflammatory changes over several spinal levels and cord compression at vertebral levels L3, L4.

Investigations

- When clinical suspicion is high, immediate spine imaging should be pursued.
- Gadolinium-enhanced MRI is the procedure of choice (Figure 7.5); the whole spine should be imaged when possible.
- Depending on institutional resources and clinical features, CT, CT myelography, or myelography may be pursued.

Management

- Multiple consultants, including neurosurgery and infectious disease, are often involved to formulate a treatment plan.
- Surgical decompression remains a mainstay of treatment.
- Blood cultures and abscess cultures should be obtained.
- CT aspiration and antibiotic therapy may be a treatment option in selected cases.
- Antibiotic therapy should be broad spectrum and include coverage for *Staphylococcus* and MRSA.
- Reasonable initial antibiotic choices would include coverage for *Staphylococcus*, MRSA, and Gram-negative coverage.
- Postoperative patients developing spinal epidural abscess should receive additional antistaphylococcal coverage.

Other CNS Infections

Many other organisms may infect the central nervous system with a spectrum of clinical presentations including headache, meningitis, seizures, altered mental status, and cognitive impairment. A few deserve special emphasis because they are encountered with some frequency in clinical practice. Often these diagnoses are discovered in the investigation of other more common processes.

Neurocysticercosis

Neurocysticercosis is a parasitic infection by the pork tapeworm *Taenia solium*. Pigs serve as a reservoir and transmission is fecal-oral between humans. It is endemic in some areas of the world, and because of immigration patterns, neurocysticercosis is being seen more commonly in the United States.

Pathophysiology

- The parasite enters many different tissues and is often destroyed by the individual's immune system.
- Should entry into the CNS occur, the immunologically shielded CNS allows the parasite to develop further and create cysts.

History and Physical Examination

Two clinical syndromes are common presentations:

- Seizures—a cyst or cysts may serve as an epileptogenic focus.
- Headache (with or without mental status changes)—cysts may occlude the ventricular system causing an obstructive hydrocephalus.

Clinical Pearls

- Antihelminthic measures paradoxically may lead to more inflammation and a worsening of the clinical condition. Consultation is advised before initiating therapy.

Investigations

- Neuroimaging will show cystic lesions.
- Obstructive hydrocephalus may be present on neuroimaging.

Management

- Treatment is controversial.
  - Many individuals are asymptomatic and cysts are discovered with neuroimaging performed for other indications.
  - Seizures should be controlled in the usual manner.
  - Hydrocephalus will require treatment either through ventricular shunting or ventricular endoscopic fenestration.
  - Solitary large cysts may be amenable to surgical excision.

CNS Toxoplasmosis

Toxoplasmosis is caused by the intracellular protozoan parasite, *Toxoplasma gondii*. Asymptomatic infection with seropositivity ranges from about 15 percent in the population of the United States to 50 percent in some European countries.

Pathophysiology

- The protozoan parasite may infect nucleated cells of most warm-blooded animals. Felines are the definitive host. Human infection may occur from ingestion of oocytes from the soil or from ingestion of encysted meat, commonly lamb or pork. It may also be acquired by handling cat feces or contaminated soil (or cat litter).
- Most clinical toxoplasmosis results from reactivation of latent infection in patients with immunosuppression from HIV/AIDS or malignancies.
- CNS toxoplasmosis encephalitis is the common terminology, though the pathophysiology is that of small abscesses with lesions in the basal ganglia and at gray-white matter interface.
- Congenital toxoplasmosis from transplacental infection may occur if women have a primary infection during pregnancy. The triad of congenital toxoplasmosis is chorioretinitis, hydrocephalus, and intracranial calcifications (not discussed further here).

History and Physical Examination

- Headache, confusion, with or without fever, is the typical presentation. If the patient has HIV and a low CD4 count, CNS toxoplasmosis is a likely diagnosis.
- Focal neurologic deficits may be present, reflecting the locations of the focal lesions in the brain.
- Seizures may be a presentation.

Clinical Pearls

- Patients with HIV infection and CD4 counts of less than 100 are at high risk for reactivation of latent toxoplasmosis
- Extracerebral toxoplasmosis syndromes include chorioretinitis, pneumonitis, and, less commonly, involvement of the spinal cord, musculoskeletal system, heart, liver, and other organ systems.

Investigations

- Serologic testing for IgG antibody may not distinguish active disease from latent infection.
- Detection of antigen for *T. gondii* by ELISA testing indicated acute infection.
- The organism may be recovered from brain abscess aspiration or biopsy.

- Cranial CT typically shows multiple ring-enhancing lesions. The nodules are common in the basal ganglia, but they may be scattered throughout the brain. Surrounding edema is often present.
- MRI techniques will also demonstrate the lesions.
- The asymmetric target sign is characteristic, with ring-enhancing abscess within abscesses.

Management

- Administer anticonvulsants if seizures have occurred.
- Steroids are recommended if there is midline shift on CT scan or significant mass effect on CT.
- Combination antibiotic treatment is recommended:
  - Pyrimethamine with sulfadiazine, with leucovorin calcium (folinic acid) to ameliorate pyrimethamine hematologic adverse effects.
  - Alternatively, use pyrimethamine (with leucovorin) and clindamycin, if patient cannot tolerate sulfdiazine.
- Clinical improvement often precedes radiologic improvement.
- Prophylactic treatment:
  - For patients with HIV who are seropositive and have CD4 counts of less than 100.
    - Trimethoprim-sulfamethoxazole is the recommend regimen.
    - Alternative prophylactic regimens include dapsone with pyrimethamine.

Lyme Disease

CNS Lyme disease is caused by the spirochete, *Borrelia burgdorferi*.

Pathophysiology

- Lyme disease is transmitted by the bite of a deer tick—Ixodes scapularis (in most parts of the country). The tick must be attached for > 48 hours to successfully transmit the disease.
- Once the organism is in the skin, it can proliferate and spread either by direct extension, or via the lymphatics and bloodstream.
- Despite the invasiveness, there is very little inflammation.
- Both the peripheral nervous system and the CNS can be involved.

History and Physical Examination

- A history of early Lyme disease with the characteristic rash—erythema migrans—is often present. Although the classic bull's-eye rash may be present, a large homogenous erythema is more common. Other presentations include:
  - Meningitis with lymphocytic predominance
  - Cranial nerve weakness (particularly the seventh nerve, which may be bilateral)

- Radiculitis
- Myelitis, cerebellitis, and encephalitis
- Other clinical syndromes associated with Lyme disease are more controversial.

Clinical Pearls

- The patient should have objectively identified Lyme disease and objective abnormalities of the nervous system to make this diagnosis.
- In most patients with CNS involvement, the rash is no longer present.
- Although early Lyme disease is highly seasonal, CNS involvement usually presents weeks to months after the tick bite.
- A full two-thirds of patients will not give a history of tick bite.

Investigations

- Serologic testing may be problematic.
  - For CNS involvement, demonstration of anti-*Borrelia burgdorferi* antibody in the serum or CSF should be performed.
  - ELISA testing is recommended as an initial step.
  - Western blot testing should follow in equivocal or positive specimens.
  - Cross-reactivity does occur with other diseases caused by spirochetes, such as syphilis, but other testing should delineate these disorders.

Management

Treatment recommendations vary, but commonly include a third generation cephalosporin (ceftriaxone or cefotaxime) given intravenously for 14–28 days. The longer course is recommended by some because of occasional relapses. This should be managed in consultation with a neurologist or infectious diseases specialist.

Rocky Mountain Spotted Fever

Rocky Mountain spotted fever (RMSF) is not usually classified as a CNS infection, but may, at times, produce a clinical picture of a toxic-appearing patient with headache and altered mental status. It is a tick-borne illness and deserves special mention because of response to tetracycline. Between 1996 and 2000, the number of cases of Rocky Mountain spotted fever in the United States fluctuated between 400 and 600 cases per year. Between 2000 and 2002, the number of cases steadily increased to approximately 1,500 cases per year. Most cases are in the south Atlantic and south central states. RMSF is a systemic infection and rickettsia cause inflammation in the vascular endothelial cells with widespread vascular lesions in many organ systems. Vasculitic or purpuric rash is frequently present, and many different

153

organ systems are affected. CNS symptoms may cover the spectrum, ranging from headache to coma.

Pathophysiology

- Etiologic agent: *Rickettsia rickettsii*
- Rod-shaped bacterium with cell wall
- Tick borne – by the larger dog tick (*Dermacentor* species)
- Invades vascular endothelial cells causing vasculitis

History and Physical Examination

- Incubation time is 2–14 days.
- Patient presents with fever, severe headache, myalgias, nausea, vomiting, renal failure, pulmonary edema.
- CNS (brain or spinal cord) is involved in 20–25 percent of cases.
- Stupor, coma, seizures, papilledema, ataxia, delirium, or vertigo may be presenting signs.
- Focal deficits may be present and include aphasia, hemiplegia, and cranial nerve abnormalities
- 20 percent of patients present with meningeal signs and photophobia.
- 90 percent of patients present with rash, usually diffuse, including palms and soles, and the rash may be maculopapular (initially) or purpuric (later).

Clinical Pearls

- Most patients will present with a picture of nonspecific viral-type syndrome with prominent headache and myalgias.
- The rash does not typically appear till the third day of the illness and never appears in 10–15 percent of patients.
- A few patients may present with a meningitic picture or other CNS abnormalities.
- Suspect these infections with a history of tick-bite or in summer seasons when ticks are active, although one-third of patients will not give a history of a tick bite.

Investigations

- CBC may show leukocytosis (with left shift) but more commonly, the WBC is normal; thrombocytopenia is common.
- Chemistries may show hyponatremia or elevated liver function profile.
- CSF may be normal.
- Lymphocytic or neutrophilic pleocytosis (1–200 wbc), protein elevated in 30–50 percent (19–236 mg/dl) of patients.
- Imaging may show edema, white matter lesions, or small hemorrhages.
- Focal infarction on CT has been reported in rare cases.

Management

- Tetracycline (500 mg q.i.d.) or Doxycycline (100 mg b.i.d.) for 7–10 days; doxycycline should be given IV in patients with severe illness.
- Chloramphenicol or ciprofloxacin are of unclear or inconsistent efficacy.
- Because the diagnosis is rarely proven initially, the treatment must be started on the suspicion of RMSF.

Human Ehrlichiosis (Note: newer nomenclature is "Anaplasmosis")

- Ehrlichiosis also presents as a febrile flu-like illness and may cause headaches and irritability. It is also a tick-borne illness. The organism attacks the white blood cells. Two infectious agents produce almost clinically indistinguishable syndromes, human monocytic ehrlichiosis (HME), and human granulocytic ehrlichiosis (HGE).

Pathophysiology

- Etiologic agent is a small, Gram-negative, obligate intracellular rickettsia.

- *Ehrlichia chaffeensis* causes human monocytic ehrlichiosis (HME, vector is *Amblyomma americanum*).
- *Ehrlichia phagocytophilia* causes human granulocytic ehrlichiosis (HGE, vector is *I. scapularis*).
- Ehrlichiosis was recognized as a new human disease in 1986.
- HME is found in southeastern and southcentral United States.
- he is found in Wisconsin, Minnesota, Connecticut, California, Maryland, New York, Florida.
- Most common April–Sept., Males>Females, >60 years old.

Clinical Pearls

- A summer flu presentation with leukopenia, thrombocytopenia, and mild elevation of transaminases is a classic clinical picture.
- Ehrlichiosis is caused by an organism that is not susceptible to cephalosporins or beta-lactam antibiotics.

History and Physical Examination

- Not all patients will give a history of tick bite.
- Generalized febrile illness with rash, severe headache, malaise, nausea, vomiting, rigors.

Investigations

- Pancytopenia with leukopenia, thrombocytopenia, and often anemia
- Liver function profile is often abnormal.

- Clumps of intracytoplasmic organisms ("morulae") may be present on examination of the peripheral blood smear, more commonly in HGE.
- PCR: Unknown sensitivity and specificity
- If CSF is sampled, lymphocytes may be present, sometimes polymorphonuclear leukocytes (PMNs), which are often in the 5–100 WBC range.
- CSF protein may be normal or moderately elevated.

Management

- A tetracycline is the drug of choice as with RMSF; ill-appearing patients with possible ehrlichiosis should be treated empirically with IV doxycycline.
- Other treatment is supportive.

Suggested Readings

Attia J, Hatala R, Cook DJ, Wong JG. The rational clinical examination. Does this adult patient have acute meningitis? *JAMA.* 1999;282:175–181.

Darouiche RO. Spinal epidural abscess. *N Engl J Med.* 2006;355:2012–2020.

Garcia HH, Del Brutto OH. Neurocysticercosis: updated concepts about an old disease. *Lancet Neurol.* 2005;4:653–661.

Halperin JJ. Nervous system Lyme disease. *Vector Borne Zoonotic Dis.* 2002;2:241–247.

Kupila L, Vuorinen T, Vainionpaa R, Hukkanen V, Marttila RJ, Kotilainen P. Etiology of aseptic meningitis and encephalitis in an adult population. *Neurology.* 2006;66:75–80.

Miner JR, Heegaard W, Mapes A, Biros M. Presentation, time to antibiotics, and mortality of patients with bacterial meningitis at an urban county medical center. *J Emerg Med.* 2001;21:387–392.

Osborn MK, Steinberg JP. Subdural empyema and other suppurative complications of paranasal sinusitis. *Lancet Infect Dis.* 2007;7:62–67.

Osman Farah J, Kandasamy J, May P, Buxton N, Mallucci C. Subdural empyema secondary to sinus infection in children. *Childs Nerv Syst.* 2009;25:199–205.

Sendi P, Bregenzer T, Zimmerli W. Spinal epidural abscess in clinical practice. *QJM.* 2008;101:1–12.

Thomas KE, Hasbun R, Jekel J, Quagliarello VJ. The diagnostic accuracy of Kernig's sign, Brudzinski's sign, and nuchal rigidity in adults with suspected meningitis. *Clin Infect Dis.* 2002;35:46–52.

Tunkel AR, Glaser CA, Bloch KC, et al. The management of encephalitis: clinical practice guidelines by the Infectious Diseases Society of America. *Clin Infect Dis.* 2008;47:303–327.

Uchihara T, Tsukagoshi H. Jolt accentuation of headache: the most sensitive sign of CSF pleocytosis. *Headache.* 1991;31:167–171.

van de Beek D, de Gans J. Should adults with suspected bacterial meningitis receive adjunctive dexamethasone? *Nat Clin Pract Neurol.* 2008;4:252–253.

van de Beek D, de Gans J, McIntyre P, Prasad K. Steroids in adults with acute bacterial meningitis: a systematic review. *Lancet Infect Dis.* 2004;4:139–143.

van de Beek D, de Gans J, McIntyre P, Prasad K. Corticosteroids for acute bacterial meningitis. *Cochrane Database Syst Rev.* CD004405; 2007.

van de Beek D, de Gans J, Spanjaard L, Weisfelt M, Reitsma JB, Vermeulen M. Clinical features and prognostic factors in adults with bacterial meningitis. *N Engl J Med.* 2004;351:1849–1859.

Chapter 8

Selected Cranial and Peripheral Neuropathies

Magdy H. Selim and Jonathan A. Edlow

159

Introduction

Chapter 8 deals with isolated cranial nerve lesions, anatomically grouped polycranial neuropathies, and selected peripheral nerve lesions. The cranial nerve nuclei lie in the brainstem and exit at various locations. Cranial nerve abnormalities within the brainstem are almost always associated with other neurological symptoms and signs. It is possible for a cranial nerve nucleus to be damaged without adjacent tissue involvement, but this is exceptionally rare. Because the anatomy of the brainstem is so crowded with other structures—long tracts traveling down to the spinal cord or up to the brain—central cranial nerve lesions are almost always associated with other findings and, therefore, are very useful for localization.

Sometimes, multiple cranial nerve palsies are found in a given patient. Several anatomic syndromes are seen. Nerves that traverse the cavernous sinus for example (the third, fourth, sixth, and first two divisions of the fifth) can be affected together, again helping with localization. Tumors in the region of the cerebello-pontine angle can also cause grouped cranial nerve findings that suggest both the location of the lesion and its differential diagnosis.

It is important to note that other times, polycranial neuropathies are not anatomically grouped. One example of this is in facial nerve palsy, in which case, occasionally, other non-contiguous cranial nerves may also be affected. Also, patients with an indolent infectious meningitis that tends to affect the base of the brain (e.g., Lyme, Cryptococcus), can have dysfunction of several cranial nerves that do not localize anatomically (other than that they all traverse the subarachnoid space at the base of the brain). Still another example would be patients with myasthenia gravis, who may have various cranial nerve findings that do not localize (e.g., a right sided ptosis and a left medical rectus palsy).

Finally, there are some peripheral nerve lesions that are sufficiently common to be included in this chapter. Patients with these problems will sometimes fear that they are having a stroke or other serious neurological condition, and the clinician that can make the diagnosis of a peripheral lesion will be able to alleviate their anxieties.

Cranial Nerve Neuropathies

Third Nerve Palsy

Anatomic notes

- The nuclei of the third nerve lie in the midbrain; because the third nerve innervates four different extra-ocular muscles (EOMs), there are four distinct subnuclei (see Chapter 2—diplopia)

- Note that there is a second nucleus—the Edinger Westphal nucleus—that is close in location and that houses the parasympathetic fibers, which constrict the pupils, that travel with the third nerve.
- The parasympathetic fibers are peripherally located within the nerve and tend to be on the supero-lateral surface (thus vulnerable to external compression).
- The third nerve traverses the subarachnoid space and enters the cavernous sinus.
- As the third nerve exits the sinus, it enters the orbit via the superior orbital fissure.

Innervations

- The third nerve innervates four of the six extra-ocular muscles (EOMs)– the medial, superior, and inferior rectus muscles, and the inferior oblique.
- It also innervates the levator palpebrae.
- Parasympathetic fibers that travel with the internal carotid artery also lie peripherally along the supero-lateral portion of the third nerve.

Presentation

- There are two common types of third nerve palsy—pupil-involving and pupil-sparing.
- A complete pupil-involving third nerve palsy presents with:
  - The affected eye "down and out" in the neutral gaze
  - Ptosis
  - The pupil fixed and dilated
- A complete pupil-sparing third nerve palsy presents with:
  - The affected eye "down and out"
  - Ptosis
  - The pupil normal in size and reactivity
  - Headache or facial pain is often a retro-orbital pain or pressure.
- This pain may be worse in patients with masses compressing the third nerve.
- Diplopia (sometimes referred to as "blurred vision" by patients.
- Ptosis.
- Dilated, nonreactive or poorly reactive pupil.

Clinical Pearls

- The most common cause of pupil-involving third nerve palsy is a cerebral aneurysm, usually of the posterior communicating artery; these aneurysms often have not ruptured, so the headache may not be the classic thunderclap headache seen in SAH.

- The pathophysiology of pupil-sparing third nerve palsy is microvascular infarction from small vessel disease of the *vasa nervorum*. These patients tend to be older, diabetic, hypertensive, and smokers.
- In patients who do not have a complete third nerve palsy, this distinction between external compression and microvascular infarction is much less clear.
- In patients with pupil-involving third nerve palsy, MRI can be falsely negative in cases of small aneurysms (<5 mm).
- In patients whose ptosis is severe, they may not complain of diplopia because they are only seeing out of the nonptotic eye.
- In patients with asymmetric pupils, it is not always the large one that is abnormal. Generally it is the pupil that reacts less or does not react at all (to light) that is the abnormal one.
  - *If the abnormal pupil is small* because of abnormality in dilatation, then the pupillary size difference will become greater in the darkness (as in Horner's). Patients with Horner's syndrome have miosis (small pupil) on the affected side.
  - *If the abnormal pupil is large* because of an abnormality in constriction, then the pupillary size difference will become greater in light.

Investigations

- Neurological or neurosurgical consultation is recommended in all patients with third nerve palsy.
- In most patients, some form of cerebrovascular imaging is recommended—CTA, MRA or (less and less frequently) catheter angiography.
- Some patients with otherwise typical pupil-sparing third nerve palsy may not need angiography; however, close clinical follow-up is recommended. Even if such a patient is discharged from the ED without an in-person consultation, urgent neurology follow-up should be arranged.

Management

- For pupil-sparing third nerve palsy, control of vascular risk factors (smoking and alcohol cessation and blood pressure control) is important. These lesions usually resolve over 6–12 months.
- For pupil-involving third nerve palsy, treatment is directed at the underlying cause. If the cause is aneurysmal, either surgical clipping and endovascular coiling can be used depending upon the morphology of the aneurysm. Reports suggest that even in patients treated endovascularly, the symptoms tend to resolve.
- Simple measures, such as an eye patch to prevent diplopia or tape to maintain the ptotic lid elevated can also help.

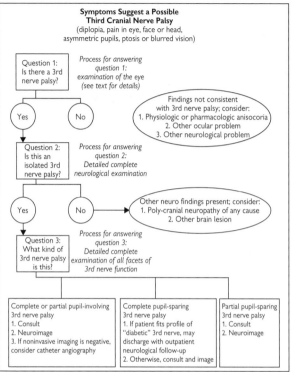

Symptoms Suggest a Possible Third Cranial Nerve Palsy
(diplopia, pain in eye, face or head, asymmetric pupils, ptosis or blurred vision)

Question 1: Is there a 3rd nerve palsy?

Process for answering question 1: examination of the eye (see text for details)

Yes — No

Findings not consistent with 3rd nerve palsy; consider:
1. Physiologic or pharmacologic anisocoria
2. Other ocular problem
3. Other neurological problem

Question 2: Is this an isolated 3rd nerve palsy?

Process for answering question 2: Detailed complete neurological examination

Yes — No

Other neuro findings present; consider:
1. Poly-cranial neuropathy of any cause
2. Other brain lesion

Question 3: What kind of 3rd nerve palsy is this?

Process for answering question 3: Detailed complete examination of all facets of 3rd nerve function

Complete or partial pupil-involving 3rd nerve palsy
1. Consult
2. Neuroimage
3. If noninvasive imaging is negative, consider catheter angiography

Complete pupil-sparing 3rd nerve palsy
1. If patient fits profile of "diabetic" 3rd nerve, may discharge with outpatient neurological follow-up
2. Otherwise, consult and image

Partial pupil-sparing 3rd nerve palsy
1. Consult
2. Neuroimage

Figure 8.1 Algorithm for an approach to patients with third nerve palsy.

Figure 8.1 provides an approach to the management of patients with possible 3rd cranial nerve palsy

Sixth Nerve Palsy

Anatomic Notes

- The nuclei of the sixth nerve lie in the pons.
- After exiting the brainstem, the sixth nerve has the longest intra-cranial course of any of the cranial nerves, making it more vulnerable to changes in ICP, especially high pressures.
- For this reason, a sixth nerve palsy is not a localizing finding.

Innervations

- The sixth nerve innervates the lateral rectus muscle,

Presentation

- Diplopia (horizontal—the two images are side by side).

- Other systemic or neurological symptoms may be present due to the underlying cause; headache is common.
- Look for papilledema.

Clinical Pearls

- Because most cases of sixth nerve palsy are due to elevated ICP, the presence of a sixth nerve palsy is not localizing; in fact, it is frequently referred to as a "falsely localizing" sign.
- There are two common causes of sixth nerve palsy: inflammation and changes in ICP.
- When doing an LP in this situation, always measure the opening pressure.
- Causes due to changes in ICP include the following:
  - Any cause of elevated ICP, including pseudotumor cerebri and cerebral venous sinus thrombosis
  - Sixth never palsy is occasionally seen in spontaneous intracranial hypotension
- Causes due to inflammation include chronic or basilar meningeal infection or infiltration (such as Lyme, TB, or Cryptococcus, carcinomatous or lymphomatous meningitis).
- Demyelinating disease
- Thyroid ophthalmopathy
- Myasthenia gravis

Investigations

- Utilize brain imaging (CT or MRI) to find a mass lesion.
- If the imaging is negative, do an LP.
- In addition to the standard CSF tests, consider testing for TB, Lyme Cryptococcus, syphilis, tumor cells, oligoclonal bands, and others according to specific patient epidemiological factors. Also, thyroid function tests should be considered.
- Neurology consultation should be strongly considered in all of these patients.

Management

- The management of the sixth nerve palsy is a function of the underlying cause; for example, a posterior communicating aneurysm would be clipped or coiled, whereas Lyme meningitis would be treated with antibiotics.

Seventh Nerve Palsy

Anatomic Notes

- The nucleus of the seventh nerve lie in the pons, close to the sixth nerve nucleus.

Table 8.1 Selected Causes of Peripheral Seventh Nerve Palsy		
Cause	Agent or Mechanism	Comments
Idiopathic "Bell's palsy"	Probably HSV infection	A small percentage of these patients may have other co-existent cranial neruopathies
Ramsay Hunt syndrome	HZV	Vesicles in external ear canal
Lyme disease	*Borrelia burgdorferi*	Often bilateral, ask about the skin rash – erythema migrans
Guillain-Barré syndrome	Inflammatory polyneuropathy	Can be bilateral
Sarcoidosis	Granulomatous inflammation	Can be bilateral
Sjogren's syndrome		
HIV infection	Infection v inflammation	
Parotid tumors	Direct compression	
Head trauma	Direct trauma/ compression to nerve in bony canal	

- The main nerve picks up other branches responsible for secretions from the lacrimal and salivary glands, taste on the anterior two-thirds of the tongue via the chorda tympani.

Innervations

- The seventh nerve innervates the muscles of facial expression.
- The muscles in the lower face receive innervation from upper motor neurons in the cortex from only the contralateral hemisphere; whereas the muscles to the upper face receive innervation from both cerebral hemispheres.
- The seventh nerve innervates the stapedius muscle in the ear (which normally dampens down sound intensity in the ear).
- The seventh nerve is also responsible for tears and saliva.
- The seventh nerve also supplies sensation to a small portion of the external auditory meatus. (Table 8.1)

Presentation

- Because of the pattern of innervation, one must distinguish between a peripheral (lower motor neuron) and a central (upper motor neuron) seventh nerve palsy. Bell's palsy typically refers to idiopathic lower motor neuron seventh nerve palsy. Ischemic stroke is the most common case of a central facial palsy.

- The hallmark of seventh nerve palsy is unilateral facial weakness.
- Patients with a peripheral seventh nerve palsy have weakness of the entire side of the face, including the facial muscles on the forehead.
- Patients with a central seventh nerve palsy have preserved forehead muscles; it is important to note, however, that some patients with central seventh nerve palsy (those with a pontine or insular infarct, can mimic a peripheral seventh nerve palsy.
- Ear pain or retroauricular fullness.
- Hyperacusis (from stapedius dysfunction).
- Decreased tears (leading to dry eyes and corneal trauma).
- Altered taste (dysgeusia) due to chorda tympani involvement.

Clinical Pearls

- Typical Bell's palsy is almost always unilateral; bilateral seventh nerve palsy suggests Lyme disease, sarcoidosis, Guillain-Barré syndrome or, if fluctuating, myasthenia gravis.
- Idiopathic seventh nerve palsy is much less common in children; therefore, always consider Lyme disease in pediatric patients, especially if the epidemiologic context is right.
- Vesicles in the external ear canal suggests the Ramsay-Hunt syndrome (causes by HZV).
- Ask, "Close your eyes tightly," to test the upper facial muscles (with upper face involvement, the eyes will not close tightly due to orbicularis oris involvement.
- Ask, "Show me your teeth," to test the lower facial muscles.
- Ptosis is NOT due to seventh nerve palsy.

Investigations

- The investigations will depend entirely on which spectrum of the differential diagnosis that is being considered; for example brain imaging will be needed if a central cause is present.
- For typical Bell's palsy, no imaging is indicated, although if done, CT will almost always be normal and MRI may show inflammation of the seventh nerve or the geniculate ganglion.
- Specific testing (for Lyme disease or Guillain-Barré syndrome or other specific causes (nonidiopathic seventh nerve palsy) will depend on which of those disease processes one is testing for. For example, consider a chest x-ray and angiotensin converting enzyme level if sarcoidosis is possible.
- Strongly consider secondary causes in children, whose underlying risk of idiopathic disease is much lower; especially consider Lyme disease

- For cases due to Lyme disease, controversy exists about the necessity of doing an LP; in European cases, patient outcomes were equivalent with oral antibiotics regardless of whether CSF pleocytosis was present.
- Neurology consultation is not necessary for routine cases but close follow-up is.

Management

- The management of the seventh nerve palsy will depend on the underlying cause.
- In idiopathic causes, the practice standards of the American Academy of Neurology suggest that oral corticosteroids is probably effective, antivirals are possibly effective, and that there is insufficient evidence to recommend surgical decompression.
- If steroids and antiviral agents are used, many practitioners use a 7–10 day course.
- Eye protection is important. During the day, patients should use saline drops and at night, an ointment, such as Lacrilube to avoid corneal drying and abrasions.

Eighth Nerve Palsy

Anatomic Notes

- The eighth cranial nerve is actually two separate nerves: the cochlear and the vestibular.
- Both originate in the lower pons and exit in the region of the cerebello-pontine angle.
- They then exit the skull via the internal auditory canal.

Innervations

- The cochlear nerve innervates the cochlea responsible for hearing.
- The vestibular nerve innervates the peripheral vestibular apparatus.
- These two nerves can be affected together or separately.

Presentation

- Acute cochlear nerve palsy presents as a sensori-neural type hearing loss (see Acute Hearing Loss in Chapter 2—Presenting Symptoms) for more details.
  - Acute onset of diminished hearing
  - If there is partial hearing loss, sounds may appear distorted or "harsh."
  - Fullness or pressure in ear
  - Tinnitus
  - Some patients will also have some dizziness or vertigo.

- Acute vestibular neuronitis presents as an acute peripheral vestibular syndrome (see Dizziness in Chapter 2 – Presenting Symptoms for more details)
- Abrupt onset of dizziness, usually vertigo (the illusory sense of motion) lasting hours to days.
- Although symptoms will be worsened by head movement, they are constant and not primarily brought on by change in head position.
- Nausea, vomiting, and mild to moderate gait instability are common.
- Horizontal, unilateral, non-direction changing nystagmus is common.

Clinical Pearls

- The head thrust test (also called the head impulse test) is an easily performed bedside test to help distinguish cerebellar infarction from vestibular neuritis (see Figure 8.2).

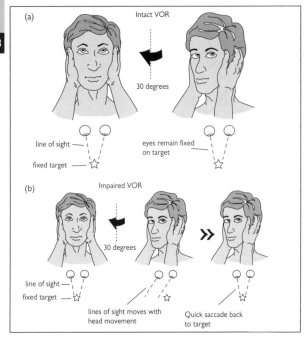

Figure 8.2 (a) A graphic of a patient with an intact vestibulo-ocular reflex (VOR). (b) A patient with an impaired VOR. The impaired reflex is found in patients with peripheral lesions (e.g., vestibular neuritis) while the normal VOR is seen in patients with cerebellar stroke.

- Direction changing nystagmus is almost always central.
- The vast majority of cases of acoustic schwannoma do not exhibit dizziness (even when they do have hearing loss or tinnitus) because the lesion is such a slow-growing one.
- In the Weber test, patients with acute sensori-neural hearing loss will hear louder in the good ear, whereas in a conductive hearing loss (e.g., cerumen impaction, or a middle ear effusion), they will hear better in the bad ear.
- Some cases of patients with acoustic schwannoma will have an acute presentation of hearing loss.
- Occasional patients with acute unilateral hearing loss, with or without tinnitus (especially if they have vascular risk factors), can have an ischemic infarct of the anterior inferior cerebellar artery.

Investigations

- Cochlear nerve
  - Careful ENT exam including external canal, tympanic membrane, Weber and Rinne tests
  - Urgent ENT evaluation
  - Audiogram
  - MRI with gadolinium if acoustic schwannoma is a possibility (not necessarily emergently)
- Vestibular nerve
  - In some cases, such as younger patients without vascular risk factors for stroke who have a positive head thrust test, no further testing is needed to make the diagnosis.
  - In other cases (a negative head impulse, or an older patient with many risk factors for stroke), brain imaging is indicated, MRI being preferable.
  - In this latter group of patients, remember that CT scan is much less sensitive for brain ischemia and infarction, especially so in the posterior fossa.
  - If there is significant ambiguity in the diagnosis, then urgent ENT or neurology consultation is recommended.
  - If acute cerebellar infarction is a possibility, emergent neurology consultation should be strongly considered.

Management

- Cochlear nerve:
  - For acute sensori-neural hearing loss, limited data suggest steroids improve outcomes. Although a Cochrane review showed that steroids are "unproven," many authorities use a 10–14 day tapering course or prednisone.

- Some ENT practitioners use intratympanic steroid injection though the data for this intervention are extremely limited.
- Data for antiviral agents are limited.
- Consider noise protection with ear muffs or plugs.
- Scuba diving should be avoided in patients who have had an acute sensori-neural hearing loss.

• Vestibular neuritis:

  - Consider a course of steroids, typically for approximately two weeks.
  - Antiviral agents have not been shown to help, but some clinicians still use them with the same rationale as for seventh nerve palsy.
  - A "labyrinthine suppressant," such as meclizine, dimenhydrinate, or lorazepam may be useful; however, the duration should not exceed several days to enhance recovery
  - Consider vestibular exercises.

Anatomically Grouped Cranial Nerve Syndromes

When more than one cranial nerve is affected simultaneously, two general possibilities should be considered. The first is that there is an anatomic reason for the distribution of nerves involved. Examples include a lesion of the cavernous sinus or cerebello-pontine angle in which the nerves involved are due to the focality of the lesion. The other possibility is that the distribution of nerves involved is not due to a localized anatomic cause. Examples of the latter group would be the polycranial neuropathy that occurs in approximately 10 percent of Bell's palsy cases, or a patient with cryptococcal meningitis with a sixth nerve palsy and an acute sensori-neural hearing loss due to inflammation at the base of the brain. Botulism would be another rare example.

When multiple nerves are involved for anatomic reasons, there is obvious localizing value, but in addition, certain differential diagnoses are suggested. The more common anatomically grouped polycranial neuropathies are discussed in this section (Table 8.2):

Cavernous Sinus Thrombosis

Anatomy

- The cavernous sinus is a venous sinus through which the carotid artery and several cranial nerves pass. The venous inflow is from the superior and inferior orbital veins.
- The pituitary gland lies medial to the cavernous sinus.

Table 8.2 **Anatomically Grouped Cranial Nerve Syndromes***	
Cavernous sinus syndrome	Third, fourth, sixth, and V¹ and V² divisions of the fifth nerves; internal carotid artery
Superior orbital fissure syndrome	Third, fourth, sixth, and the V¹ division of the fifth nerve
Orbital apex syndrome	Same as above PLUS the optic nerve
Cerebello-pontine angle syndrome	Fifth and eighth nerves (both components), cerebellum
Jugular foramen syndrome	Ninth, tenth, and eleventh nerves
Internuclear ophthalmoplegia	See section on Diplopia

*All of these syndromes can present with various combinations of the nerves listed in the table.

- The sphenoid sinus lies inferior to the cavernous sinus.
- Besides the carotid artery, the third , fourth , the two divisions of the fifth, and the sixth cranial nerves traverse the cavernous sinus.

Presentation

- Because of the various components of the cavernous sinus, the nerves affected can be variable.
- Diplopia is the most common symptom (66 percent) followed by peri-orbital pain (35 percent).
- Complete ophthalmoplegia is present in less than 20 percent of cases.
- Facial paresthesias can occur from fifth nerve involvement.
- Some patients have proptosis with or without chemosis.
- If the underlying process is infectious, fever may be present.
- Five percent of cases are bilateral.
- In one form of the cavernous sinus syndrome—the Tolosa Hunt syndrome—pain is more predominant and its cause is sterile inflammation.

Clinical Pearls

- Initially, one of the four cranial nerves that traverse the cavernous sinus may be affected.
- In one series of 136 cases, tumors caused 63 percent of cases; of these, pituitary adenoma accounted for over half, and meningiomas were only slightly less common.
- In the same series, vascular causes (aneurysms and cavernous-carotid fistulae) accounted for 20 percent, and the Tolosa Hunt variety accounted for another 13 percent of cases. Tolosa-Hunt is

a sterile granulomatous inflammatory process that can involve the cavernous sinus or the orbit.

- Thrombosis due to infection or hypercoagulable state, accounted for only a single case.
- Cavernous sinus thrombosis.
- Because the sympathetic fibers join the sixth nerve within the cavernous sinus, a Horner's syndrome with a sixth nerve palsy localizes to the cavernous sinus.
- When the cause of cavernous sinus syndrome is thrombosis, *Staph aureus* is the most commonly isolated organism, followed by *Strep pneumo* and fungal species.

Investigations

- Diagnostic testing will be a function of the specific differential diagnosis in any given case. MRI (with or without contrast but with venous phase) is the preferred imaging test.
- CT scan, usually with contrast, can be used initially if MRI is not available.
- In rare cases, CSF analysis may be useful, but it is not routine.

- Neurology consultation should be strongly considered in all cases.
- Get blood cultures in cases thought to be infectious.

Management

- The treatment is directed at the underlying cause.

Superior Orbital Fissure and Orbital Apex Syndromes

Anatomy

- The superior orbital fissure is an elongated passage from the middle fossa into the orbit. It is located at the medial sphenoid ridge between the lesser and greater wings of the sphenoid. Cranial nerves three, four, six and the first division of five traverse the superior orbital fissure.
- The optic nerve traverses the orbital canal that lies just medial to the superior orbital fissure.
- The orbital apex is where the contents of these two holes in the skull come together.
- The ophthalmic artery and superior ophthalmic vein also enter the orbit at the orbital apex.

Presentation

- Eye pain
- Diplopia

- Facial paresthesias of the forehead
- Decreased corneal sensation
- Proptosis and chemosis
- The principle difference between the superior orbital fissure syndrome and the orbital apex syndrome is visual symptoms due to optic nerve involvement.

Clinical Pearls

- Careful testing of vision and the three divisions of the fifth nerve are important to distinguish between lesions in the cavernous sinus, superior orbital fissure, and orbital apex.
- Visual acuity abnormalities (optic nerve involvement) usually implies a surgical emergency to decompress the orbit.
- Tolosa-Hunt syndrome can involve the orbit and can respond dramatically to high- dose steroids; pain often resolves more rapidly than the physical findings.
- Neurology consultation should be strongly considered in all cases.

Investigations

- Thin cut orbital CT or MRI
- Neurology consultation
- Usually, ophthalmology consultation (always if there is decreased visual acuity).

Management

- The management is a function of the underlying etiology and location of the lesion.
- Visual impairment from orbital pathology often requires emergency decompressive surgery.
- In some cases, high-dose steroids are used (Tolosa-Hunt syndrome).

Cerebello-Pontine Angle Syndrome

Anatomy

- This triangular space is bounded by the undersurface of the cerebellum, laterally by the pons, and superiorly by the petrous ridge of the temporal bone.
- The fifth through eighth cranial nerves are most commonly are affected.

Presentation

- 95 percent have hearing loss, although it is so insidious that many patients are not aware of it.
- 60 percent have tinnitus; this tends to subside as the hearing loss becomes complete.
- About 60 percent will have vestibular nerve involvement, but, again, because of the insidious nature of the lesion, clinically important dizziness is unusual.
- Less than 20 percent of patients have facial numbness or dysesthesia (fifth nerve)
- A small minority have facial weakness (seventh nerve).

Clinical Pearls

- The vast majority of cerebello-pontine angle lesions are tumors.
- Of these, 80–90 percent are acoustic shwannomas, and the majority of the remainder are meningiomas.
- 10 percent of patients with neurofibromatosis have tumors in the cerebello-pontine angle; consider examining the skin for café au lait spots.
- Occasionally, patients with acoustic shwannomas will present with an acute sensori-neural hearing loss.

Investigations

- MRI is the imaging test of choice.
- CT scan, usually with contrast, can be used initially if MRI is not available or contra-indicated for some reason.
- Use audiograms to measure hearing loss.
- Neurology and/or ENT consultation should be strongly considered.

Management

- The treatment is directed at the underlying cause; surgery is the usual therapy.
- Stereotactic radiotherapy and proton beam therapy have also been used.
- Occasional cases may be observed over time; this is up to the discretion of the specialist and patient.

Jugular Foramen (Vernet's) Syndrome

Anatomy

- The jugular foramen lies at the junction of the middle and posterior cranial fossae.
- Cranial nerves nine, ten, and eleven traverse this foramen.

Presentation

- Dysphagia
- Loss of taste on the posterior one-third of the tongue
- Hoarseness
- Weakness of the trapezius and sternocleidomastoid muscles

Clinical Pearls

The most common causes of the jugular foramen syndrome are metastatic tumor, schwannoma, meningiomas and glomus tumors.

Investigations

Both CT and MRI are used to image this area.

Management

The treatment is directed at the underlying cause.

Peripheral Neuropathies

Radial Nerve Palsy

Anatomic notes

- The radial nerve is made up of various components of the brachial plexus and follows the humerus in the spiral groove.

Innervations

- The motor functions of the radial nerve are wrist and finger joint extension and, forearm supination.
- One constant area of sensation is the first dorsal web-space (between thumb and index finger).

Presentation

- The classic symptoms and signs are those related to wrist drop; there is no active extension at the wrist.
- In proximal lesions, all the extensor muscles in the arm can be affected.
- There is reduced or absent sensation as already mentioned, and along the postero-lateral side of the arm.
- Triceps reflex is reduced or absent.

Clinical Pearls

- Other terms include "Saturday night palsy" (intoxicated individual falls asleep with their arm draped over a chair or car door) and "crutch palsy" (using crutches improperly or using poorly fitted crutches).

- Radial nerve palsy can be mistaken for a stroke; careful history and physical examination should be able to distinguish between the two.
- Radial nerve palsy can be seen in association with humeral fractures.
- Distally, the superficial branch at the wrist can be compressed by handcuffs or tight restraints affecting sensation to the dorso-lateral hand.
- Lead poisoning tends to affect the radial nerve.

Investigations

- No investigations are generally required because the diagnosis is usually established clinically.

Management

- Advise avoidance of the activity leading to compression.
- Treat the humerus fracture if present.
- Treat the lead poisoning if present.

Carpal Tunnel Syndrome

Anatomic Notes

- The median nerve arises primarily from the C6 and C7 roots.
- In the wrist, it passes in the carpal tunnel, along with the flexor tendons deep to the flexor retinaculum, an area subject to compression.

Innervations

- The median nerve innervates muscles represented by the mneumonic LOAF:
  - Lumbricals 1 and 2
  - Opponens pollicis
  - Abductor pollicis brevis
  - Flexor pollicis brevis (superficial head)
- One constant area of sensation is the palmar aspect of the middle finger.

Presentation

- Patients have wrist pain that often shoots distally into the fingers.
- Symptoms are often worse at night; patients will awaken feeling a need to shake their hands to relieve the pain.
- There is a decreased sensation in the second and third digits
- When asked to make a fist, the thumb and index finger do not flex, giving the appearance of gesturing upwards (sometimes called a "preacher's hand" or an "orator's hand."

- Positive Tinels's sign (worse symptoms on percussion of the median nerve at the wrist).
- Positive Phalen's sign (worse symptoms on maintenance of the wrists in forced flexion for a minute).
- Thenar atrophy in advanced cases.

Clinical Pearls

- The pains are sometimes described more like dysesthesias.
- The sensory symptoms sometimes radiate proximally up the arm rather than distally.
- The median nerve can also be compressed in the upper arm, sometimes referred to as "honeymooner's palsy."
- Consider the diagnosis of C6 or C7 radiculopathy.

Investigations

- To some extent, this will depend on the underlying cause (see Table 8.3); in the absence of an obvious cause, a thyroid stimulating hormone (TSH) and HgbA1c should be considered.
- The diagnosis of carpal tunnel can be established by nerve conduction studies.

Management

- Treat the underlying disorder.
- Utilize night wrist splints.
- Medications such as gabapentin may help with the pain.
- Consider steroid injection.
- For idiopathic cases and those for which there is no particular treatment, the flexor retinaculum can be released surgically.

Femoral Nerve Palsy

Anatomic Notes

- Portions of the L2, 3, and 4 roots make up the femoral nerve.

Table 8.3 Causes of Carpal Tunnel Syndrome
Repetitive stress injury (such as house painting, typing, etc.)
Edema and inflammation (e.g., rheumatoid arthritis)
Pregnancy and oral contraceptives
Hypothyroidism and acromegaly
Uremia
Diabetes
Amyloidosis
Wrist fracture

Innervations
(See Tables 8.4 and 8.5)
- Motor functions include hip flexion and knee extension.
- Sensation is to the medial leg and a constant area is the medial aspect of the knee.
- The femoral nerve is responsible for knee jerk.

Presentation
- Pain in the groin and anterior thigh
- Weakness of hip flexion and the knee extension
- Numbness along the medial leg

Clinical Pearls
- The nerve can sometimes be affected by pelvic trauma or retroperitoneal hematoma (or other compression at that location).
- Diabetic patients (and others with vascular risk factors) can have an ischemic femoral nerve microvascular infarction (similar to a diabetic third nerve palsy. This tends to happen in male type-2 diabetics and is sometimes called "diabetic amyotrophy" as the anterior thigh can atrophy.

Investigations
- Imaging may be necessary if there is a question of retroperitoneal pathology or root disease.

Management
- Treat of the underlying condition.
- For diabetic microvascular infarction, patients tend to improve spontaneously over 6–12 months.

Sciatica

Anatomic Notes
- The sciatic nerve is comprised mostly of the L5 and S1 roots that emerge from the lumbo-sacral plexus.
- It is most vulnerable to injury shortly after its formation.
- It gives off the tibial and common peroneal nerves.

Innervations
(see Tables 8.4 and 8.5)
- The L5 root is responsible for great toe dorsiflexion, first dorsal web space sensation.
- The S1 root is responsible for foot plantar flexion, lateral fifth toe sensation, and the ankle jerk.

Table 8.4 Quick Exam to Test for Patients with Back Pain

Root	Motor	Sensation	Reflex
L3 and L5	Extension of the knee	Medial knee	Knee jerk
L5	Dorsiflexion of the great toe	First dorsal web space of foot	none
S1	Plantar flexion of the foot	Lateral fifth toe	Ankle jerk

Table 8.5 Quick Exam to Test for Patients with Neck Pain

Root	Motor	Reflex
C5	Shoulder Abduction and elbow flexion	Biceps
C6	Elbow flexion (while semipronated)	Supinator
C7	Finger and elbow extension	Triceps
C8	Finger flexors	Finger
T1	Hand intrinsic muscles	None

Presentation

- Patients often have back or buttock pain, often from an acute herniated disc.
- Weakness in leg (depending on which root is involved (see earlier)
- Numbness in lower leg and foot

Clinical Pearls

- Although sciatica is typically due to lumbar disc disease, remember that other compressive (tumor), inflammatory (Lyme disease), and trauma (after IM injections in the buttock) can also affect the nerve.

Investigations

- The diagnosis is usually made clinically.
- Plain films are useless.
- CT scan can show the problem, but MRI is far more sensitive.
- MRI, although more sensitive, is unnecessary in the vast majority of cases and should be reserved for those cases for which surgery is planned or if a secondary cause (tumor, infection or hematoma) is being considered.

Management

- The vast majority of patients with sciatica from a disc improve spontaneously.
- Surgery, including micro-discectomy is reserved for selected cases.

Peroneal Nerve Palsy

Anatomic Notes

- The common peroneal nerve passes very superficially around the fibular neck at the knee.

Innervations

- The peroneal nerve is responsible for foot eversion and dorsiflexion.
- Sensation is the dorso-lateral foot.

Presentation

- The most common symptom and sign is the presence of foot drop; the patient has difficulty walking due to inability to dorsi-flex
- Foot drop can occur from several types of problems:
  - Injury to the dorsiflexor muscles
  - Swelling in the leg fascial compartments, causing muscle ischemia
  - Peripheral damage to the peroneal nerve (e.g., trauma, lumbar disc herniation, post-knee surgery)
  - Rarely, foot drop can be seen after a central processes.

Clinical Pearls

- The superficial location of the nerve makes it vulnerable to compression, trauma, and stretch; common causes are direct blunt trauma, thigh stockings, tight cast, or even crossing one's legs.
- In an L5 radiculopathy, foot inversion is also involved.

Investigations

- Usually the diagnosis is apparent from history and physical examination.

Management

- Once the mechanical cause is removed, most patients recover.
- A foot brace can improve symptoms while the lesion heals.

Suggested Readings

Baloh RW. Clinical practice. Vestibular neuritis. *N Engl J Med.* 2003;348(11):1027–1032.

Buracchio T, Rucker JC. Pearls and oysters of localization in ophthalmoparesis. *Neurology.* 2007;69(24):E35–E40.

Edlow JA, Newman-Toker DE, Savitz SI. Diagnosis and initial management of cerebellar infarction. *Lancet Neurol.* 2008;7(10):951–964.

Gilden DH. Clinical practice. Bell's Palsy. *N Engl J Med.* 2004;351(13):1323–1331.

Hotson JR, Baloh RW. Acute vestibular syndrome. *N Engl J Med.* 1998;339(10):680–685.

Rauch SD. Clinical practice. Idiopathic sudden sensorineural hearing loss. *N Engl J Med.* 2008;359(8):833–840.

Rucker JC, Tomsak RL. Binocular diplopia. A practical approach. *Neurologist.* 2005;11(2):98–110.

Stanton VA, Hsieh YH, Camargo CA, Jr., et al. Overreliance on symptom quality in diagnosing dizziness: results of a multicenter survey of emergency physicians. *Mayo Clin Proc.* 2007;82(11):1319–1328.

Sullivan FM, Swan IR, Donnan PT, et al. Early treatment with prednisolone or acyclovir in Bell's palsy. *N Engl J Med.* 2007;357(16):1598–1607.

Woodruff MM, Edlow JA. Evaluation of third nerve palsy in the emergency department. *J Emerg Med.* 2008;35(3):239–246.

Chapter 9

Traumatic Head Injury

Daniel C. McGillicuddy and John E. McGillicuddy

Incidence of Head Injury

Traumatic head injury accounts for over one million nonfatal traumatic brain injury (TBI) cases and 52,000 deaths in the United States per year. Traumatic brain injuries occur in a bimodal pattern; in the age group 15–24, most TBI are due to gunshot wounds or motor vehicle crashes, and in the patient population over the age of 65+, most injuries are due to falls.

Pathophysiology of TBI

Acute Primary Brain Injury

- Cell injury and death of the brain cells and vascular network due to the direct application of force.
- There is no treatment other than prevention.
- The only prevention is avoidance of injury; programs to increase automobile seatbelts and fall-prevention programs have become important functions of trauma centers.

Secondary Brain Injury

- Secondary brain injury is cellular injury that is delayed and remote from injury.
- These cells—neuron, glia, and cerebral vasculature cells—are injured by different mechanisms as compared with primary brain injury, and the injury usually occurs in a delayed fashion.
- Causes of secondary brain injury include:
  - Hypoxia
  - Hypotension
  - Hypertension
  - Brain ischemia
  - Increased intracranial pressure
- When brain cells are injured, they may begin to swell secondary to changes in the permeability of their membranes. Intracellular water accumulates resulting in cytotoxic brain edema. Swelling of the brain also may be accompanied by intracranial hemorrhage. The rigid skull has a fixed volume, and as the volume of the material inside this space—brain, cerebrospinal fluid, and blood—increases, the pressure within the skull increases. There are some compensatory mechanisms (see later), but once these are overwhelmed, intracranial pressure (ICP) can increase exponentially. In addition, the cerebral blood vessels are also injured and may respond to trauma by losing their ability to regulate cerebral blood flow (CBF) through a process

called autoregulation. Autoregulation acts to maintain a steady rate of CBF in the face of changes in arterial pressure. Loss of autoregulation may lead to critically low blood flows if systemic blood pressure falls below a mean arterial pressure of about 50 mm of mercury.

Critically low cerebral blood flow (CBF) causes cerebral ischemia, resulting in further cell membrane damage and increased intracellular fluid. Also, leakage of fluid from damaged capillaries further increases extracellular fluid. All of these factors contribute to an increasing cascade of increasing intracranial contents.

Because the skull is a fixed space, the transfer of cerebral spinal fluid to the spinal dural sac and of blood through the venous sinuses to the general circulation can compensate some of this increase in intracranial volume. However, once these shifts have been maximized, any further increase in brain edema or any accumulation of abnormal bleeding within the skull leads to a sharp increase in ICP.

Increased ICP itself affects cerebral blood flow by increasing the resistance to flow. The cerebral perfusion pressure (CPP) is determined by the difference between mean arterial pressure (MAP) and the ICP representing the resistance at the outflow end. This is expressed as the equation:

$$CPP = MAP - ICP$$

Normal cerebral blood flow is 50 cc's per 100 grams of tissue per minute. This steady flow is ensured by the autoregulation of the cerebral vascular tree. When MAP decreases, the intracerebral vessels dilate, and when MAP increases, the cerebral vascular vessels constrict. This varies the resistance in the system and thus stabilizes flow. When CPP drops below 50 mm Hg, or when autoregulation fails, as in head trauma, cerebral blood flow becomes pressure passive, and flow varies directly with the CPP. This is why severely increased ICP or severely decreased MAP will cause a marked decrease in cerebral blood flow. When cerebral blood flow drops below 20 cc per 100 grams per minute, brain cell membrane function breaks down, cell functions cease, and cells begin to die and swell.

Finally, the brain is very dependent on oxygen and cannot function more than a few minutes on anaerobic metabolism. Thus, systemic hypoxia is devastating to brain function and to the viability of brain tissue. Very short periods of hypoxia can have a major deleterious effect on eventual brain function. Hypercarbia can also cause cerebral arterial dilation, which can increase ICP.

Thus, prevention of secondary causes of brain injury must include maintenance of an adequate cerebral perfusion pressure both by avoiding hypotension (systemic) and by lowering ICP. It is also critical to maintain excellent oxygenation and ventilation.

Clinical Signs and Symptoms of TBI

The history of injury may often be elicited, but occasionally patients are found down without a history. Patients who have suffered a traumatic brain injury can be alert, awake, and appearing well or they may be moribund and comatose. There is almost always the history of injury, although this is not always available. Patients will usually have signs of injury to the head, neck, or trunk, such as contusions or lacerations, but they must be searched for carefully.

Symptoms

- Headache
- Blurry Vision
- Amnesia
- Tinnitus

Physical Signs

- Transient or persistent loss of consciousness
- Depressed or disturbed mentation, lethargy, and coma
- Scalp laceration
- Cranial nerve palsy
- Battles Sign (ecchymosis at the mastoid process from skull fracture)
- Raccoon Eye (orbital ecchymosis from skull fracture)
- Hemiparesis, paralysis, or focal weakness
- Otorrhea or rhinorrhea of clear cerebral spinal fluid (CSF)
- Hemotympanum (blood in the middle ear)
- Vomiting
- Ataxia
- Seizure

Initial Management and Evaluation of the Head-Injured Patient

This should be a rapid assessment to evaluate acute life threats. The physician must methodically assess a patient's stability, and determine if interventions are required prior to a full and complete assessment. One must pay close attention to the ABCs (Airway, Breathing, and Circulation) in any trauma patient. Attention should be paid to maintaining an appropriate and stable airway, to assure adequate breathing, and to assess circulation and obtain IV access. Upon completion of the ABCs, attention should be turned to the neurological status of the patient, while periodically reassessing the airway, breathing, and circulation. This is vital because, as mentioned earlier, even brief episodes of hypotension or hypoxia can lead to worse outcomes by causing preventable secondary brain injury.

Patients with significant head injury will often need their airway actively managed to prevent aspiration from vomiting, and to oxygenate and ventilate the comatose patient. Have a low threshold to intubate the head-injured patient. After completion of the primary survey (ABCs), the priority shifts to looking for other injuries including neurological ones. One typically uses the Glasgow Coma Score. The Glasgow Coma Scale (GCS) is a commonly used 15-point scale to assess a patient's neurological status after head injury. A score of 14 or higher is considered a minor head injury; 9–13 is a moderate head injury, and 8 or below is a severe head injury.

Box 9.1 Glasgow Coma Scale: Add the Best Result to get Total Score. Range 3–15

187

Eye Opening
- Spontaneous 4 pts
- To speech 3 pts
- To pain 2 pts
- No response 1 pt

Verbal Response
- Alert and oriented 5 pts
- Disoriented 4 PTS
- Nonsensical speech 3 pts
- Unintelligible or moaning speech 2 pts
- No speech 1 pt

Motor Response
- Follows commands 6 pts
- Localized pain 5 pts
- Withdraws from pain 4 pts
- Decorticate (Flexor) posturing 3 pts
- Decerebrate (Extensor) posturing 2 pts
- No Response 1 pt

Investigations

- Examine pupil size, response to light, extraocular movements, and any gaze palsy or ptosis.
- Compare the two sides of the body for motor strength by voluntary response or response to pain. Pay close attention to lateralizing differences as they may suggest a spinal cord injury or an extra-axial brain hematoma or ICH.
- Examine the scalp for active bleeding or signs of open skull fracture. Scalp bleeding can be massive and will occasionally be responsible for a patient's hypotension. It should quickly be managed as part of the ABCs. A pressure dressing or skin staples can adequately manage most scalp lacerations during the acute phase. Wear a glove when probing the laceration.
- Examine the face for signs of mid-facial instability or oral trauma that could predict a difficult intubation.
- Examine the tympanic membranes for signs of hemotympanum, which is often associated with basilar skull fractures.
- Examine the head for 'raccoon eyes' and nasal CSF leakage.

Box 9.2 Do not forget

Maintain C Spine precautions with inline immobilization and a cervical collar if available.

Maintain C Spine precautions when rolling the patient to examine their back, and while assessing for secondary injuries.

Perform a complete trauma assessment as patients with head injuries often have associated injuries to the neck, thorax, or extremities.

Airway Management

Active airway management is often needed in the head-injured patient.

Indications for Early Intubation

- GCS < 8
- Respiratory or cardiac failure/arrest
- Persistent vomiting
- Evidence of hypoxia or airway obstruction
- Severe uncontrollable agitation
- Severe polytrauma
- Anticipated future course. Examples include
1. Patient will need to be intubated for some other reason (such as going to the operating room for repair of another injury).

2. Patient requires transport to a different facility (in which case intubation may be more difficult during transport).
3. Patient may have prolonged imaging outside the emergency department (and also be in a place not conducive to rapid airway management).

Intubation of the Head-Injured Patient

Cervical spine injuries are often associated with TBI, so remember to keep the patient in a cervical collar or inline stabilization up to the point of intubation. During intubation the collar can be removed while maintaining in-line cervical stabilization (usually by a specific individual not involved in the intubation) to prevent cervical spine movement. Once the endotracheal tube has been confirmed and secured, a rigid cervical collar should be put back in place.

Rapid sequence intubation (RSI) with a short-acting paralytic and induction agent is the standard intubation technique for most trauma patients. The specific medications are beyond the scope of this chapter, but some practitioners also administer "pre-medication" in the minute(s) prior to the paralytic and induction agents in order to blunt the rise in ICP induced by laryngoscopy. In exceptional patients, severe facial injuries may preclude oral intubation, in which case a surgical cricothyroidotomy should be performed to assure airway security.

The important principles to remember are to avoid hypoxia, hypercarbia, and hypotension, because these factors can significantly increase the morbidity and mortality of the head-injured patient.

Finish the Primary and Secondary Survey

After assessing and securing the airway as necessary and prior to moving the patient from the resuscitation bay for diagnostic imaging, ensure that a complete primary and secondary surveys have been completed.

Box 9.3 Assure

- Breathing: Hypoxia leads to increased morbidity and mortality and must be avoided. Supplemental oxygen is used as needed to achieve oxygen saturations greater than 95 percent; adequate ventilation to avoid hypercarbia is also important although excessive hyperventilation (to a PaCO2 < 32) is to be avoided.
- Circulation: Keep a systolic BP > 90 mm Hg, until an ICP monitor can be inserted if needed. Then aim for a CPP of 60–70 mm Hg.
- Disability: Note focal neurological deficits. Maintain adequate cervical spine precautions with a rigid cervical collar or in-line stabilization. Whenever possible, perform and document the neurological exam prior to administration of medications for RSI.
- Exposure: Fully examine the patient for injuries to the neck, thorax, extremities, and be sure to roll the patient to examine the back for injuries.

189

Imaging of the Head-Injured Patient

Patients that are severely injured enough to warrant endotracheal intubation or those with a GCS ≤ 8 should undergo CT imaging of the head if they are stable enough to undergo CT scans. Several studies have tried to address the issue of when to image the less severely injured patient. Controversy exists regarding if and when CT scans should be done on the less-severe head injuries. Following are some suggestions about when a brain CT scan may be indicated.

Who Should Get a Head CT after Trauma?

This is a suggested list of those who should likely get a CT scan of the head after trauma. **NB: This list is not all inclusive and many other patients with blunt head injury not included in this list will likely need imaging as their clinical course dictates.**

- Those with GCS < 14
- Those who are intoxicated or have altered mental status
- Those with focal neurological deficit
- Those who are anticoagulated (especially with warfarin)
- Those with a serious mechanism of injury (fall from height, high speed motor vehicle crash, etc.)
- Those with loss of consciousness or amnesia who posses one of these risk factors:
  - Age > 60
  - Headache
  - Vomiting
  - Seizure
  - Persistent anterograde amnesia
  - Drug or alcohol intoxication
  - Visible trauma above the clavicles

Specific Injuries

Extra-Axial Injuries

These are injuries to the scalp, skull, and extraparanchymeal portions of the calvarium.

Scalp Laceration

There are five layers to the scalp; skin, subcutaneous tissue, epicranial aponeurosis (galea), loose areolar tissue, and the pericranium.

Lacerations through these tissues can lead to significant blood loss and cosmetic defect. Direct pressure to control the bleeding followed by local wound infiltration using lidocaine with epinephrine will usually allow for adequate control of bleeding. The wound should be explored to evaluate for retained foreign bodies, skull fractures, and galeal or muscle lacerations, because deep scalp lacerations will often need deep suturing prior to skin closure. Remember to use sterile technique while closing lacerations and that adequate irrigation is a primary method to reduce wound infection. Sometimes a defect in the galea can mimic a depressed fracture.

Skull Fractures

Fractures to the skull can sometimes be difficult to detect because the suture lines may resemble fractures, and the skull has variable anatomy. Skull fractures are usually qualified by location, type, and whether the fracture is compound (i.e., skin breakage over fracture site). All patients with skull fractures should undergo CT scan imaging of the brain to evaluate for associated injuries.

There are two types of skull fractures:

- Linear skull fractures involve both the inner and out tables of the skull (except in some fractures involving the paranasal sinuses). Depressed skull fractures may also occur. Most depressed skull fractures will undergo operative repair. If there is an associated skin laceration, then prophylactic antibiotics are often indicated because these are treated like compound fractures.

- Basilar skull fractures involve the anterior skull base with the sphenoid, ethmoid, and frontal bones, as well as the temporal bone, and they will often extend into the auditory canal (Figure 9.1). They will often have associated pneumocephalus or fluid in the mastoid air cells as signs of fracture. Common physical exam finding of basilar skull fractures include: battles sign (contusion over mastoid process), CSF otorrhea or rhinorrhea, hemotympanum, or periorbital ecchymosis. Patients with basilar skull fractures should be evaluated by a neurosurgeon. There is a small risk of associated meningitis with basilar skull fractures, and prophylactic antibiotics that cover typical skin flora and also possess adequate CSF penetration may be recommended; however, their indiscriminate use can select out resistant organisms. Otorrhea almost invariably stops, and prophylactic antibiotics are virtually never necessary for this injury. It is important to remember **not** to place nasogastric tubes or nasal feeding tubes in patients with basilar skull fractures.

Epidural Hematoma

These injuries usually arise after a blow to the head has disrupted the middle menningeal artery located in the parietal temporal bone. These patients will often have a transient loss of consciousness,

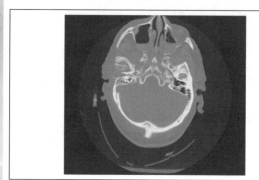

Figure 9.1 Basilar skull fracture.

followed by a period of lucidity and than a rapid decline from increased intracranial pressure. The patients are often described as "talk and decline".

Epidural hematomas are due to arterial bleeding and, therefore, expand rapidly. On CT scans they appear as hyperacute fluid (white) with a lenticular shape that does not usually cross suture lines. The blood collects between the brain and the dura, and exerts a lateral and often downward pressure on the brain and brainstem. All but the smallest of epidural hematomas will require surgical repair, often with an open craniotomy to gain control of arterial bleeding. While there is some emerging data that patients with small (<1 cm) epidural hematomas can be observed without surgical intervention, the standard of care would still dictate neurosurgical consultation and evaluation.

Patients with epidural hematomas require emergent management, neurosurgical consultation for consideration of operative repair, and very close ICU level monitoring for those who do not undergo surgery. (Figure 9.2)

Subdural Hematomas

These injuries arise from injury to the bridging veins or from cortex lacerations and their associated arterial bleeding, and they can result in bleeding between the dura and the arachnoid. These injuries usually arise from a blunt force mechanism; however, they can arise without direct head trauma (such as rapid acceleration or deceleration). Patients with brain atrophy or coagulation problems (elderly, alcoholics, hemodialysis) are at a higher risk of developing subdural hematomas with minimal to no trauma. Acute traumatic subdurals are vastly different than chronic subdurals; the bleeding in acute subdural hemorrhages can be due to laceration of the cerebral cortex,

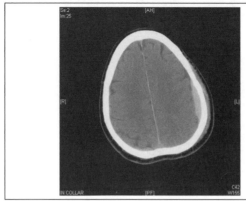

Figure 9.2 Epidural hematoma.

and they can be arterial in nature, whereas the bleeding in chronic subdurals or low energy injuries is often venous in nature.

In contrast to the rapid onset of bleeding seen with epidural hematomas, subdurals that are venous in nature typically have a more indolent time of onset and progression. They are typically graded as acute, subacute, and chronic, based on CT density of the extra-axial blood. These will often coexist in the same patient (i.e., chronic subdural from remote trauma now with acute bleeding from fall). See Figures 9.3, 9.4, and 9.5.

Like any head injury, the presenting symptoms can be vague, such as subtle change in mental status, mild headache, or vomiting, or they can be extreme, such as hemiparesis or coma. Subdural hematomas on CT scan will appear as concave-shaped extra-axial fluid collections that cross suture lines and that will usually cause lateral compression. Because patients with brain atrophy are at higher risk for sudural hematomas, there can be a significant fluid collection with little to no cerebral shift or herniation.

Patients with subdural hematomas detected on CT scan should have a neurosurgical consultation and evaluation. Patients with acute and subacute subdurals will often benefit from neurosurgical intervention. Depending on the severity of their symptoms, patients with chronic subdurals can often be managed nonoperatively.

Historical data shows that patients with acute subdural hematomas benefit from early operative intervention with a significant decrease in mortality if undergoing surgery within four hours. Patients with traumatic subdurals often have underlying serious brain injuries, and the venous bleeding and oozing can be more difficult to control. Also, the patients are often older. For all of these reasons, the morbidity

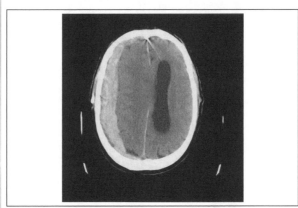

Figure 9.3 Subdural acute.

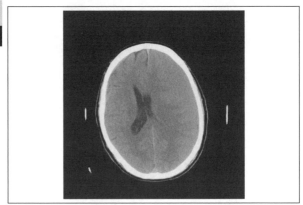

Figure 9.4 Subdural subacute.

and mortality of acute subdurals is typically higher than that of acute epidural hematomas.

Traumatic Subarachnoid Hemorrhage

Traumatic subarachnoid hemorrhage (tSAH) can result from blunt head injuries. These injuries are detected by CT or MRI scanning. Blood is found in the subarachnoid space usually located near the site of trauma. Because patients with aneurysmal SAH can fall and sustain head trauma, it can be difficult to discern the cause of subarachnoid bleeding.

The location of the bleeding—isolated near the circle of Willis vs. peripheral near a site of trauma—plus the history (headache

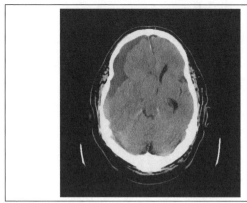

Figure 9.5 Chronic subdural.

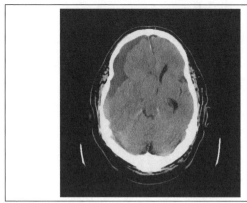

prior to fall) can help point the clinician toward the correct etiology. However, there is no foolproof method by noncontrast CT imaging to prove the cause of bleeding (aneurysm rupture vs. trauma), and some form of angiography may be necessary.

Patients with tSAH should have a neurosurgical consultation and evaluation. Because the data about the utility of nimodopine's effectiveness in preventing vasospasm in tSAH are unclear, the use of this medication should be left to the discretion of the consulting neurosurgeon. The presence of a tSAH portends a significant increase in morbidity and mortality, therefore, these patients should be admitted to the hospital for serial neurological exams and possible serial imaging, as exam dictates. See Figure 9.6.

Intra-Axial Head Injury

Intra-axial injuries pertain to the brain parenchyma. These are direct injury to the brain cells with disruption of the blood-brain barrier.

Cerebral Contusions

Cerebral contusions arise from direct trauma to the brain parenchyma. These are some of the most common injuries. They are usually found in the frontal lobe, the temporal lobes, and the occipital lobes. These injuries are often found in pairs, that is, a coup and counter-coup injury. The coup portion of injury occurs over the area of direct trauma, and the counter-coup injury typically occurs on the opposite side of the brain. These injuries result from the mobility of the brain within the calvarium, resulting in the transmission of the force vector to the opposite side of the brain and inducing injury by the mechanism of the brain hitting the inner table of the skull.

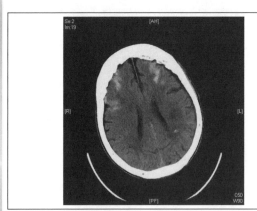

Figure 9.6 Traumatic subarachnoid.

Contusions can have a hemorrhagic portion at time of injury or can progress to hemorrhagic transformation hours to days later. These injuries are often located in the cortex, putting the patient at risk for development of seizure disorders.

These injuries can rapidly expand, especially if the patient is anticoagulated. Furthermore, due to the nature of these injuries one should carefully look for an underlying skull fracture.

Patients with cerebral contusions or hemorrhages should have a neurosurgical consultation and evaluation. Efforts to reduce intracranial pressure, such as elevating the head of bed to 30 degrees, ensuring that there are no constrictive collars or bandages around the neck, prevention of vomiting with anti-emetics, and correction of coagulopathy are all recommended. These patients should be admitted to the hospital for serial neurological exams and consideration of repeat neuron-imaging, as the clinical exam dictates.

Diffuse Axonal Injury

Diffuse axonal injury (DAI) is a result of shearing force on the axons. This is typically a result of rapid deceleration injuries (i.e., fall from height, motor vehicle crash, motor cycle crash, assault, shaken baby syndrome).

These patients will often present in a comatose state. The initial head CT can be unremarkable; however, often there will be punctuate hemorrhages in the deep structures of the brain (internal capsule, corpus callosum, or near third ventricle) (Figure 9.7).

DAI is an example of primary brain injury. It is graded as mild, moderate, or severe. In mild DAI, the coma usually lasts 6–24 hours, and leaves the patient with mild neurological deficits. Moderate DAI coma lasts longer than 24 hours and leaves the patient with motor

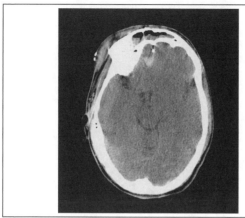

Figure 9.7 Diffuse axonal injury.

and cognitive deficits. Severe DAI is similar to moderate DAI but with associated autonomic instability.

All treatment modalities currently in use are directed at treating the secondary complications of DAI, such as seizures or increased intracranial pressure. Patients with DAI clearly need a neurosurgical consultation, ICU admission, and consideration of intracranial pressure monitoring.

Cerebral Herniation Syndromes

The end result of many moderate to severe TBI is the development of elevated ICP. As edema or blood collects within the strict volume confines of the calvarium, the pressure rises. As this pressure rises, the brain parenchyma is compressed and moved laterally, downward, or upward, depending on the location of injury/swelling or bleeding, leading to several stereotyped brain herniation syndromes.

Symptoms of these herniation syndromes are similar to all TBI: vomiting, change in mental status, headache or lethargy. Some signs of herniation syndromes include hemiparesis or quadraparesis, decreased responsiveness, dilatation of one or both pupils, papilledema, or progressive motor posturing.

Herniation Syndrome Types

- Uncal Herniation: The temporal lobe herniates through the tentorium. Usually results in contralateral hemiparesis and ipsilateral pupil dilatation due to compression of the third cranial nerve

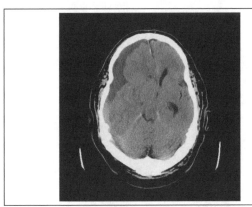

Figure 9.8 Subfalcine herniation.

- Subfalcine Herniation (Figure 9.8): This is a lateral herniation. Neurological symptoms can vary.
- Cerebellar tonsillar Herniation: This type occurs when cerebellar tonsils herniate through the foramen magnum. This will compress the brainstem, which can lead to respiratory arrest, and pinpoint pupils with quadraparesis.

Treatment of herniation syndromes is focused on fixing the primary cause (i.e., surgical repair of epidural hematoma), reducing ICP, and preventing hypotension and hypoxia.

Post Diagnosis/Secondary Management

As in all emergency cases, attention is first directed toward the ABCs of management. Once a patient's airway has been deemed to be stable or is controlled, breathing and oxygenation are sufficient, and circulation and IV access have been obtained, one can begin to focus on the management of the diagnosed injury.

This section will deal with the treatment of problems related to TBI.

Increased Intracranial Pressure

ICP is normally in the range of 10–20 mm Hg. Elevated ICP is diagnosed when the pressure exceeds 20–25 mm Hg or 20 cm of H_2O. The diagnosis of elevated ICP can be suggested by CT scan finding (i.e., obliteration of basilar cisterns, obstructing hydrocephalus, etc.); however, the true diagnosis of elevated ICP can only be made with ICP bolt monitors or intraventricular drains.

Both of these pressure monitoring modalities can be placed by a neurosurgeon.

Treatments of Elevated ICP

- Intraventricular drains: placed by neurosurgeon can drain off excess CSF and thereby decrease ICP.
  - Patients with GCS < 8 with abnormal CT scan have > 50 percent incidence of elevated ICP. Those with normal CT have a lower incidence of elevated ICP (15 percent). AANS/BTF recommends placement of an ICP monitoring or intraventricular drainage device for patients with either a GCS < 8 with abnormal CT or patients with a normal CT and atleast 2 of the 3 following high-risk criteria (age > 40 years; SPB < 90 mmHg and any motor posturing).
- Elevate of the head of bed to 30 degrees.
- Ensure the any C-spine collar or other devices are not compressing the neck.
- Administer anti-emetics to prevent vomiting.
- Mannitol and osmotic diuretic will reduce ICP while transiently increasing blood pressure and improving CPP. A delayed effect of mannitol is a diuresis, which can lead to hypotension and electrolyte abnormalities.
- Mannitol dose: 0.25 gm/kg to 1 gm/kg bolus dosing.
- Hyperventilation can reduce ICP by lowering the partial pressure of carbon dioxide, which in turn leads to vasoconstriction and reduces cerebral blood flow. This reduced blood flow can lead to a reduction in ICP; however it can also lead to cerebral ischemia. The current recommendations are for **mild** hyperventilation to a PCO2 of 30–35; anything lower can lead to cerebral ischemia.
- Hypertonic saline is currently being studied as another modality to decrease ICP. The data to date has been mixed, and its use should be at the direction of a consulting neurosurgeon.
- Hemicraniectomy with removal of part of the calvarium has been shown to occasionally be successful in relieving elevated ICP in cases resistant to other measures.

Seizure Prophylaxis

Patients who suffer TBI are at a risk of developing both early onset and delayed onset seizures. Many studies have evaluated the effectiveness of anti-epileptic medications in preventing both early and late seizures in the head-injured patient. To date, no studies have shown long-term seizure prevention by the use of anti-epileptic medications; however, there appears to be some utility in reduction of early onset (seven days or less) seizure activity if an anti-epileptic medication is used.

Risk Factors for Seizure (Citation for BTF S 83)

- GCS < 10
- Cortical contusion
- Epidural or subdural hematoma
- Intracerebral hemorrhage
- Depressed skull fracture
- Early seizure

The medication of that has been most studied is phenytoin 10–15 mg/kg IV load, no faster than 50 mg per minute. While phenytoin IV loading, the patient should be monitored for cardiac dysrhythmias and hypotension.

Blood Pressure Management

Hypotension must be avoided, as a single episode of hypotension in the head-injured patient can significantly worsen mortality. Fluid boluses to keep the systolic blood pressure greater than 90 mm hg are recommended.

- Maintain a systolic blood pressure greater than 90 mm Hg. This will help to maintain a CPP greater than 50 mm Hg if the ICP is elevated (CPP=MAP-ICP)
- Hypertension is a controversial issue without strong data to make concrete recommendations. A reasonable approach would be to leave hypertension untreated unless the MAP is greater than 120 mm Hg as a way to maintain CPP. If there is an intracranial pressure device in place, more targeted blood pressure control can be instituted with the goal of maintaining a CPP of 60–70 mm Hg.

Reversal of Anticoagulated Patient

A patient with a blunt head injury and intracranial bleeding who is anticoagulated with warfarin historically has nearly a 50 percent mortality rate. Rapid correction of the International Normalized Ration (INR) has been recommended by the American College of Chest Physicians.

Three major modalities to correct the coagulopathy are:

- Vitamin K should be given intravenously because subcutaneous vitamin K has nearly the same effect as placebo when acutely reversing elevated INR. Vitamin K will allow for the production of Vitamin K dependent clotting factors 2, 7, 9, and 10. Vitamin K will work to reverse the INR in 6–24 hours; therefore, it should **never** be the sole method of reversal of INR in an anticoagulated patient with intracranial bleeding.
  - Vitamin K IV dosing: 10 mg IV slow over 20–60 minutes for severe life- threatening bleeds.

- Be aware of the potential for anaphylactoid reaction and hypotension that is occasionally associated with IV vitamin K.

- Fresh Frozen Plasma (FFP) given in the standard dose of 2–6 units (500–1500 cc) to fully reverse a warfarin-associated coagulopathy. It may take time to obtain type-specific plasma, and it can be a significant volume load for a patient with a compromised cardiovascular system, so one should pay close attention to the patient's respiratory status when administering a large volume of FFP.

- Prothrombin Complex Concentrates (PCC): A pooled plasma derivative of vitamin K dependent factors. A single weight-based dose of PCC will reverse a patient's elevated INR in roughly 30 minutes. It is important to remember that these products should only be used in patients with warfarin- associated coagulopathies with life-threatening bleeds. They are also associated with prothrombotic complications, and a discussion with the consulting neurosurgeon is recommended when there is consideration of PCC usage. The practioner should check with the hospital blood bank or pharmacy prior to dosing the PCC because the concentrations of coagulation factor will often change by lot number. One should also co-administer FFP as most PCC have little to no factor 7.

- Recombinant activated factor IIVa is a medication that can be given along with FFP and vitamin K to correct warfarin-associated bleeding. Dosing is variable and should be discussed with a pharmacist or hematologist.

Prophylactic Antibiotics

Antibiotic therapy for open basilar skull fractures is often recommended. These antibiotics should cover typical skin flora and have adequate CNS penetration. The use of prophylactic antibiotics should be discussed with the consulting neurosurgeon.

A single small, randomized study showed that prophylactic antibiotics at time of intubation in the head-injured patient may reduce the incidence of pneumonia. Again, consideration of prophylactic antibiotic use should be discussed with the consulting neurosurgeon.

Disposition

Patients with a normal mental status, who are at their baseline function, with a negative CT scan are typically safe to discharge assuming that there are no other injuries or circumstances surrounding the head injury that would require admission.

Patients with severe postconcussive syndrome, those who have not returned to baseline mental status, or those with CT scans of the brain showing intra-axial injuries, and extra-axial injuries with the exception of simple scalp lacerations should be admitted and observed. A neurosurgical consultation should be obtained for all patients with skull fractures, extra-axial injuries (with the exception of simple scalp lacerations), and intra-axial injuries.

Key Points

- Prevent secondary injury.
- Avoid hypoxia
- Avoid hypotension.
- Avoid hypoglycemia.
- Employ early intubation for severe head injury.
- Treat elevated intracranial pressure.
- Reverse coagulopathy.
- Consult neurosurgery
- Admit patients with TBI.

Suggested Reading

Bratton SL, Chestnut RM, Ghajar J, et al. Guidelines for the Management of Severe Traumatic Brain Injury; American Association of Neurological Surgeons; Congress of Neurological Surgeons; Joint Section on Neurotrauma and Critical Care, AANS/CNS. *J Neurotrauma.* 2007;24.

Chestnut RM, Marshall LF, Klauber MR, et al. The role of secondary brain injury in determining the outcome from severe head injury. *J Trauma.* 1993;34:216–222.

De Souza M, Moncure M, Lansford T, et al. Nonoperative management of epidural hematomas and subdural hematomas: is it safe in lesions measuring one centimeter or less? *J Trauma.* 2007 Aug;63(2):370–372.

Haydel MJ, Preston CA, Mills TJ, Luber S, Blaudeau E, DeBlieux PM. Indications for computed tomography in patients with minor head injury. *N Engl J Med.* 2000 Jul 13;343(2):100–105.

Sirvent JM, Torres A, El-Ebiary M, Castro P, de Batlle J, Bonet A. Protective effect of intravenously administered cefuroxime against nosocomial pneumonia in patients with structural coma. *Am J Respir Crit Care Med.* 1997 May;155(5):1729–1734.

Tintinalli J, Kellen G, Stapczynski J. *Emergency Medicine a Comprehensive Study Guide* 6th Edition. New York: McGraw-Hill; 2004.

Vergouwen M, Vermeulen MA, Roos Y. Effect of nimodipine on outcome in patients with traumatic subarachnoid haemorrhage: a systematic review. *Lancet Neurol.* 2006 Dec;5(12):1029–1032.

Chapter 10

Intracranial Pressure (ICP) and Hydrocephalus

Scott A. Marshall, Hardin A. Pantle,
and Romergryko G. Geocadin

Disorders of ICP and Hydrocephalus May Present as Neurologic Emergencies

Abnormalities of intracranial pressure may result in pathology requiring urgent evaluation and intervention to prevent life-threatening consequences. This pathology may represent intracranial hyper or hypotension, or it may manifest as an abnormality of cerebrospinal fluid (CSF) dynamics, such as hydrocephalus. Elevated intracerebral pressure is the final common pathway for almost all pathology leading to brain death, and interventions to treat ICP may preserve life and improve neurologic function after head trauma, stroke, or other neurologic emergencies.

Cranial Vault Mechanics and CSF

The intracranial compartment can be thought of as similar to any other anatomical compartment (i.e., abdomen, forearm, etc.) This concept was put forth first by Monro and later by Kellie more than two hundred years ago. This concept helps to explain the relationship between the contents of the cranium and intracranial pressure.

Monro-Kellie Doctrine

Simply stated, this concept views the cranium as a fixed and rigid container, and any increase in one component that makes up the compartment must be offset by a similar decrease in another component (or components) of the compartment. The sum of all the components of the cranium must remain constant.

Box 10.1 Intracranial Volumes

- Brain parenchyma = 87%
- Cerebrospinal fluid (CSF) approximately 75 cc = 9%
- Blood volume (arterial: 30%, venous, capillary: 70%) = 4%

The usual first component to exit the cranium to make room for other enlarging components is CSF, which is produced at a relatively constant rate of 20 ml/hour or approximately 500 ml per day. The rate that CSF is produced is well preserved and is only reduced if cerebral blood flow approaches zero. Once the blood volume, parenchymal volume, or a new pathological

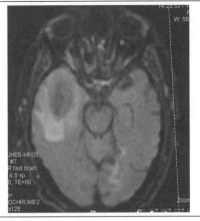

Figure 10.1 Loss of adjacent sulci exhibiting mass effect from cerebral abscess.

volume (mass, edema, hematoma) begins to enlarge, intracranial CSF is displaced into the spinal compartment. At this point, increasing mass effect then manifests radiologically as diminished appearance of the sulci or decreased ventricular size (Figure 10.1). Further mass effect will reduce blood volume, initially from the venous compartment and later from reductions in arterial blood flow. The pressure caused directly by the mass on the brain, as well as the increased intracranial pressure and decreased cerebral perfusion results in the focal deficits (hemiplegia) as well as the nonfocal neurologic manifestations such as loss of consciousness or obtundation.

Signs and Symptoms of Increased ICP

Clinically, awake and alert patients with increases in ICP will report headache, supine positioning intolerance, or other complaints, such as head pain that is worse at night and is exacerbated by Valsalva maneuvers or coughing. If the elevation in ICP is chronic, papilledema may occur. As ICP increases, nausea and vomiting may occur, along with changes in heart rate, blood pressure, and respirations. The earliest changes in vital signs may be that of tachycardia, hypertension, and hyperventilation, followed by the more classic Cushing's triad of bradycardia, hypertension, and hyperventilation. Cushing's triad represents homeostatic mechanisms to preserve arterial blood flow into a brain under pressure by increasing cerebral perfusion pressure and decreasing venous blood volume by hyperventilation.

Symptoms

- Headache, worsened with Valsalva
- Decreased visual acuity
- Diplopia
- Nausea
- Vomiting

Physical Signs

- Progressive decline in level of consciousness
- Decreased upward gaze
- Cranial nerve VI palsy
- Papilledema
- Loss of normal venous pulsations in the fundus
- Field cut or enlarged physiologic blind spot
- Alterations in vital signs

Herniation Syndromes

Herniation represents displacement of the brain parenchyma and vasculature out of their normal supratentorial or infratentorial compartments. This occurs when the compensatory mechanisms involved in maintaining ICP homeostasis are exceeded. Arterial blood flow will be limited and ischemia can ensue as part of or prior to a herniation event. Herniation syndromes produce a variety of neurologic signs and symptoms and represent a true neurologic emergency. Immediate and definitive intervention is required to prevent death or permanent neurologic disability from a herniation event.

Subfalcine, Central, and Uncal Herniation

Subfalcine herniation is lateral shift of one frontal lobe into the contralateral side, and occurs with any degree of midline shift of the cerebral hemispheres. The most common clinical manifestations are increasing lethargy and occasionally neurological deficits related to compromised flow to one or both anterior cerebral arteries (ACA). Unilateral ACA compromise classically causes weakness of the contralateral lower extremity, although involvement of the proximal arm and shoulder is reported.

Uncal, or lateral transtentorial herniation, occurs when a supratentorial mass pushes the mesial temporal lobe and uncus anteriorly and downward through the tentorial opening between the ipsilateral aspect of the midbrain and the tentorium. The third cranial nerve is located here as well. Because the pupillary constrictor fibers in the third nerve are located superficially, a dilated

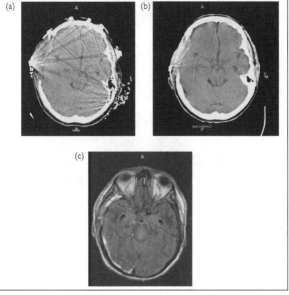

Figure 10.2 Radiographic herniation. (a) Uncal herniation, (b) duret hemorrhages of the midbrain tegmentum on HCT of the same patient 3 days later, (c) duret hemorrhages and ischemic change on FLAIR MRI of the central midbrain.

pupil may herald this phenomenon. Normally, uncal herniation results in an ipsilateral dilated pupil and contralateral hemiplegia. Sometimes, however, the pressure can compress the contralateral (to the lesion) midbrain against the tentorium, resulting in the (Kernohan's notch phenomenon). This results in ipsilateral (to the lesion) hemiparesis and contralateral (to the lesion) dilated pupil, a potentially false localizing sign. Radiographic findings of uncal herniation may be seen (Figure 10.2a) with resulting midbrain Duret hemorrhages (Figure 10.2b) and midbrain ischemia (Figure 10.2c) secondary to compromised blood flow to paramedian midbrain perforator vessels.

Central herniation is downward movement of the brainstem by pressure from the supratentorial brain components. Early findings with central herniation include cranial nerve (CN) VI palsy, manifesting as lateral gaze deficits, which can be unilateral or bilateral. Like uncal herniation, if this progresses, the clinical triad of a CN III palsy (including an ipsilateral nonreactive dilated pupil), coma, and

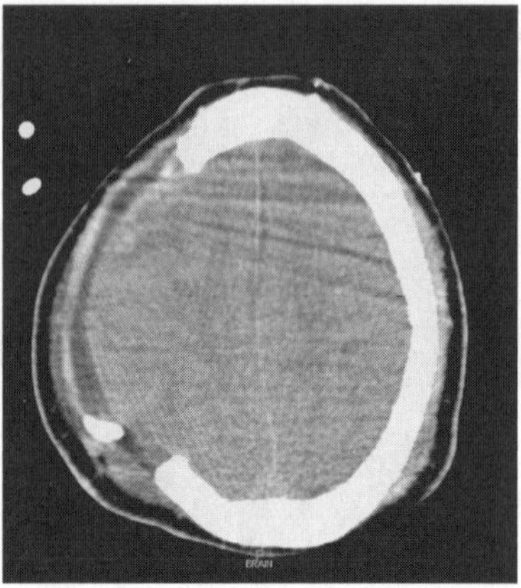

Figure 10.3 Extracranial herniation through craniectomy defect.

posturing can occur. Occasionally, unilateral or bilateral posterior cerebral artery (PCA) infarctions can occur with ongoing central or uncal herniation, due to compression of the PCA as it passes upward over the tentorial notch.

Extracranial and Paradoxical Herniation

Extracranial herniation occurs when the brain herniates through a surgical skull defect or craniectomy site (Figure 10.3). This can occur in over one-fifth of postsurgical patients with brain injury. It represents therapeutic decompression of intracranial hypertension although complications of extracranial herniation do occur and are related to laceration of cerebral cortex and vascular compromise of venous drainage (Figure 10.4). A less well described phenomenon is paradoxical herniation, which has been reported during lumbar cistern drainage in the setting of a craniectomy. Paradoxical herniation occurs when there is downward movement of brain in the setting of an overall lowered ICP. Only a handful of cases of this type of herniation are reported, although this can also occur in the setting of sodium dysregulation and hypernatremia.

Tonsillar and Upward Herniation

Tonsillar herniation occurs from downward movement of the cerebellar tonsils into the foramen magnum and compression of the lower brainstem. This type of herniation, because it does not necessarily involve arousal centers in the midbrain, may occur in an otherwise awake patient. It can result in sudden death from compression

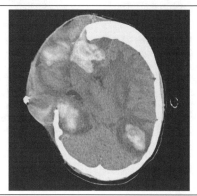

Figure 10.4 Extracranial herniation with laceration of cortex and intracerebral hemorrhage.

of medullary respiratory and blood pressure centers. Leading causes of this type of herniation are hemorrhage within the posterior fossa, edema from large cerebellar strokes, and obstruction of CSF outflow from the forth ventricle.

Upward herniation is upward movement of brain through the tentorium into the cranium. It can cause brainstem compression and can occur with excessive CSF drainage from an extraventricular drain. The clinical presentation of upward herniation, as with all herniation syndromes, can range from a slight decrease in mental status to obtundation. This can usually be prevented by avoiding overdrainage from a supratentorial extraventricular catheter.

Box 10.2 Important Points

- A posterior fossa hematoma or any significant or increasing fourth ventricular dilation, distortion, or obliteration requires urgent neurosurgical evaluation.

- Emergent extraventricular drain placement is needed to relieve obstructive hydrocephalus, but it will not relieve mass effect on brainstem.

- Large cerebellar hematomas resulting in increased ICP may have excellent neurological outcomes if surgically emergently treated.

Hydrocephalus

Hydrocephalus describes a pathologic increase in the amount of intracranial CSF relative to brain parenchyma and the intracranial blood volume. Hydrocephalus results in distortion and enlargement of the ventricular system with resultant increases in the temporal horns of the lateral ventricles, rounding of the third ventricle, and possibly enlargement of the fourth ventricle. Clinically, acute hydrocephalus is not well-tolerated, although chronic hydrocephalus may go unnoticed for some time. Acute hydrocephalus may present with headache, progressing to similar complaints and clinical findings described earlier, with increases in ICP. Hydrocephalus can be divided into three subtypes.

Communicating

Communicating hydrocephalus is the increase in CSF volume in the setting of a grossly open ventricular drainage system. This type of hydrocephalus results from the insufficient resorption or clearance of CSF from the central nervous system. This usually is caused by diminished circulation of CSF from past CNS infections (e.g., meningitis) or bleeding (e.g., SAH). Communicating hydrocephalus is treated by medical means to reduce CSF production, such as with carbonic anhydrase inhibitors or CSF removal via large volume lumbar punctures, lumbar drains, or even extraventricular drains.

Noncommunicating

Obstructive or noncommunicating hydrocephalus results from a blockage of normal CSF outflow from the intracranial compartment to the extracranial compartment. This can be due to obstruction by a tumor, hematoma, or cerebral edema anywhere along the path of CSF: lateral ventricles → foramen of Monro → third ventricle → aqueduct → fourth ventricle → central canal of the spinal cord or foramen of Luschka or Magendie. Noncommunicating hydrocephalus is treated with extraventricular drainage, and these patients should not undergo lumbar cistern drainage by lumbar puncture due to a potential for causing a herniation event with a sudden decrease in the spinal CSF pressure relative to the tonic increase in the intracranial compartment pressure.

Normal Pressure Hydrocephalus (NPH)

NPH is a potentially treatable syndrome that is one reversible cause of dementia among the elderly. It has classically been described as a triad of disorders of gait, urinary symptoms, and subcortical dementia associated with a normal or slightly elevated intracranial

CSF pressure and a communicating hydrocephalus. It is a chronic syndrome that may respond to intermittent CSF removal by lumbar puncture or lumbar drain, or most commonly with the placement of a permanent ventricular shunt.

Idiopathic Intracranial Hypertension (IIH)

IIH, also known as pseudotumor cerebri, is a disorder noted for elevations in ICP without radiographic evidence of hydrocephalus or an intracranial mass lesion. If untreated, IIH can result in unilateral or bilateral papilledema and permanent visual impairment. The classic phenotype for IIH is an obese young woman, with headaches and visual complaints, papilledema, and elevated opening pressure noted on lumbar puncture. The headaches are often described as worse upon awakening, have a throbbing quality, and are associated with photophobia. This is not unlike the symptoms reported by migraneurs, and further history is helpful to elicit further symptoms consistent with a diagnosis of IIH. These may include transient episodes of visual loss and pulsatile tinnitus. Enlargement of the physiologic blind spot is the earliest and most reported visual finding in IIH. The diagnosis of IIH should involve expert consultation with both Neurology and Ophthalmology.

Box 10.3 Risk Factors for IIH

- Obesity increases risk of IIH 20× over the general population for females ages 20–44
- Polycystic ovary disease
- Medication use including corticosteroids, cyclosporine, and tetracyclines
- Venous sinus stenosis
- Vitamin A toxicity
- Sleep apnea

A fulminate and rapidly progressive form of IIH is reported, and this may require urgent and intensive management to prevent permanent visual impairment. Severe papilledema and visual field deficits are seen early, and urgent ophthalmologic evaluation with repeated CSF drainage may be necessary until surgical intervention is available.

Box 10.4 Differential Diagnosis of IIH

- Cerebral venous sinus thrombosis
- Jugular vein thrombosis
- Superior vena cava syndrome
- Neurosarcoidosis
- Meningitis
- CNS Lupus
- Antiphospholipid antibody syndrome

Treatment of IIH

Once other conditions (see Box 10.4) with similar presentations are ruled out, management of IIH is multimodal. Weight loss is the cornerstone of therapy, and medical management should take this into account. Acetazolamide and topiramate are commonly used to decrease the production of CSF and may alleviate the headache symptoms associated with IIH. Optic nerve sheath fenestration is commonly performed, and involves creating a defect in the dural sheath surrounding the optic nerve posterior to the globe. Fenestration of the optic nerve sheath can be performed on one or both eyes, although monocular procedures may decrease visual symptoms in both eyes. Surgical means of CSF diversion include ventricular CSF shunting, which is more commonly done for refractory IIH. Bariatric surgery can also be considered in the adjunctive management of IIH. Newer interventional procedures such as dural venous sinus stenting await further study.

Intracranial Hypotension

The symptoms associated with intracranial hypotension are commonly reported as a frontal or occipital postural headache. That is, the headache is quickly relieved by lying down, and exacerbated by standing or sitting upright. This is most often a consequence of a lumbar puncture, but can occur spontaneously, due to dural leaks in the cervical or thoracic region. Intracranial hypotension can have serious consequences, including the development of subdural hematoma (SDH). If bilateral SDHs are found in a patient with no history of trauma, this condition should be ruled out. Intracranial hypotension should be remembered as an easily treatable cause of postural head pain, as the dural leak and symptoms may be quickly relieved with the placement of an epidural blood patch performed by an anaesthesiologist. Investigations include conventional MR imaging (Figure 10.5), where diffuse enhancement is

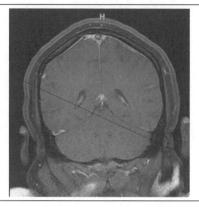

Figure 10.5 Diffuse cranial dural enhancement seen in the setting of remote spinal CSF leak.

seen of the dura mater, or CSF flow studies such as radionucleotide cisternography or CT myelography.

213

Shunt Malfunctions

Ventricular CSF shunts are not uncommon. Ventriculoperitoneal (VP), ventriculo-atrial (VA), ventriculopleural, and lumboperitoneal (LP) shunts are used for the treatment of congenital hydrocephalus, NPH, and after drain dependant hydrocephalus from trauma, hemorrhage, tumors, or stroke. Neurosurgical evaluation of a shunt is usually needed if there is a suspicion of undershunting or overshunting, infection, seizures, or otherwise when CSF is needed in a patient with a shunt in place.

Undershunting arises when a shunt drains CSF at a suboptimal rate and will present similarly to a patient with clinical hydrocephalus, with complaints of headache, diplopia, seizures, nausea, and vomiting. *Overshunting* is seen when excessive CSF is drained, and will present with postural headache (increased headache intensity when in the upright position) or other signs of intracranial hypotension, possibly including seizures or focal neurologic signs due to SDH. Either condition may be readily apparent on brain imaging. If either case is suspected, neurosurgical evaluation is warranted, and initial interventions to medically reduce ICP may be considered in the case of undershunting. Awareness of the potential for hematoma formation (SDH) with overshunting must be recognized, as discussed earlier with intracranial hypotension.

For evaluation of the patency of the shunt, the consulting neuro-surgeon will request a "shunt series" of radiographs, which includes AP and lateral skull films, and chest and abdominal x-rays (depending on the placement of the shunt). The purpose of the shunt series is to rule out disconnection, kinking, or migration of the shunt conduit. A noncontrast CT of the head is also usually indicated, and will allow for assessment of ventricular volume. CSF should only be obtained by trained personnel via aspiration of the shunt reservoir and a sample of fluid sent for analysis, depending on the clinical circumstances. Other situations that may arise with patients with a shunt in place are abnormal fluid collections along the path of the shunt, which may represent abscess. Also concerning is the development of endocardi-tis associated with infectious seeding of the heart due to meningitis in the presence of a VA shunt or peritonitis from a VP shunt.

Cerebral Edema and Elevated ICP

Types of Cerebral Edema

Cerebral swelling or edema can complicate many intracranial path-ologic processes including neoplasia, hemorrhage, trauma, autoim-mune disease, hyperaemia, or ischemia. There are essentially three types of cerebral edema:

- Cytotoxic edema is associated with cell death and failure of ion homeostasis (Figure 10.6).
- Vasogenic edema is associated with breakdown of the blood-brain barrier (BBB) (Figure 10.7).

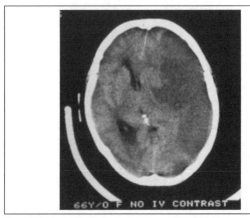

Figure 10.6 Cytotoxic edema.

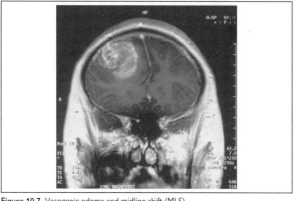

Figure 10.7 Vasogenic edema and midline shift (MLS).

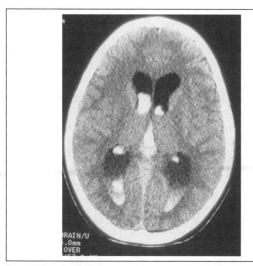

Figure 10.8 Hydrostatic edema.

• Hydrostatic edema is associated with hydrocephalus and increased tension across the ependyma of CSF containing structures (Figure 10.8).

Cytotoxic edema results from energy failure of a cell from hypoxic or ischemic stress and subsequent cell death. Intracellular swelling occurs and results in the CT and MR appearance of edema of both gray and white matter, usually in the distribution of a vascular or borderzone territory after a stroke. Vasogenic edema represents breakdown of the blood-brain barrier most radiographically prominent in the white matter, and is more likely to be associated with neoplasia or cerebral abscess. In reality, cerebral edema from many different processes usually exhibit a combination of vasogenic and cytotoxic edema. Interstitial or hydrostatic edema, also called transependymal flow, is radiographically seen with hypodense areas surrounding the ventricular system and is associated with increased CSF volume or pressure.

Treatment of Cerebral Edema

The treatment of cerebral edema involves treating the underlying cause. In cytotoxic edema, osmotic therapy with mannitol and hypertonic saline may not reduce edema in the lesion itself, but may reduce the volume of normal brain allowing for some increased margin of safety. Steroids are of no benefit in cytotoxic edema due to stroke, and may be harmful in the setting of brain trauma. Surgical treatment of cytotoxic edema with hemicraniectomy may be therapeutic. Vasogenic edema responds to steroids and surgical resection of the lesion, and may also benefit from osmotic therapy with mannitol or hypertonic saline. Hydrostatic edema is treated surgically with CSF removal or shunting, and it is treated medically with agents to decrease production of CSF.

Mass Lesions, Cerebral Abscess, and Tumors

When a CNS tumor, primary or metastatic, is found on imaging, any evidence of vasogenic cerebral edema or midline shift can be treated with high dose steroids. Dexamethasone, 4–20 mg IV every four to six hours may be needed, depending on the degree of edema. However, the use of steroids should be avoided before a biopsy is performed if there is high suspicion that the tumor could be a lymphoma, because steroids could alter the biopsy results, making the diagnosis difficult. Glycemic control and gastric ulcer prophylaxis should be remembered when starting high-dose dexamethasone. Advanced CNS imaging, including contrast enhanced MRI with diffusion imaging, will help differentiate CNS neoplasia from abscess, which is often difficult on CT imaging (Figure 10.9).

If MR is contraindicated, contrast-enhanced CT may be of utility (Figure 10.10). Seizure prophylaxis should be considered when a new diagnosis of cerebral tumor or abscess is made, and neurosurgical consultation should be obtained.

Broad spectrum antibiotics including anaerobic coverage should be started immediately upon clinical confirmation of a cerebral abscess, with cultures of sputum, urine, and blood obtained prior, if possible. The decision to obtain CSF in the setting of a cerebral abscess is

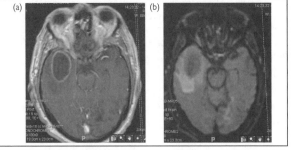

Figure 10.9 MRI appearance of cerebral abscess. (a) MR post contrast T1 weighted imaging of cerebral abscess. (b) MR fluid attenuated inversion recovery sequence (FLAIR) of cerebral abscess.

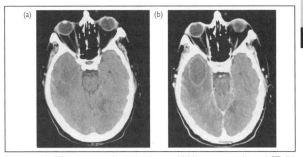

Figure 10.10 CT appearance of cerebral abscess. (a) Noncontrast enhanced CT. (b) Contrast enhanced CT.

made on a case-by-case basis, based on the degree of edema, and if any concern for increased ICP exists, then antibiotics are not delayed while debating if obtaining CSF fluid for analysis and cultures is justified. Often, a remote lesion is found on pan-body CT imaging, and this site may be amendable for direct CT-guided aspiration to help narrow antimicrobial therapy (see Chapter 7: CNS Infections).

Management of an Acute ICP Elevation

Goals for ICP

The goal for ICP management in patients with elevations in ICP is to maintain a normal intracranial pressure of less than 18 –20 cmH$_2$O or 15 mmHg. Elevations over 25 mmHg are associated with poor outcomes in trauma, and interventions should be aimed at reducing ICP to less than this level. One must keep in mind the relationship between cerebral perfusion pressure (CPP), based on mean arterial pressure (MAP) and ICP.

$$CPP = MAP - ICP$$

Many interventions to decrease ICP may also have systemic effects on peripheral hemodynamics and the lowering of MAP, thus decreasing CPP. The maintenance of a CPP of at least 60 mmHg is strongly recommended for patients with severe neurologic injury.

Elevated ICP must first be suspected before it can be treated. If a patient presents with neurologic findings, from headache to obtundation, increased ICP may be playing a role. In the initial evaluation of a neurologic emergency, an ICP monitor will not be in place to guide therapy, and thus clinical exam and radiographic studies will provide the initial information to diagnose and treat this condition. Although routine head CT should be obtained early in the management, it should not substitute for an appropriate, focused physical examination.

The ABCs

If a clinical syndrome of cerebral herniation is present, then quick action is needed to reduce morbidity and mortality. Management starts with the ABCs. As in any emergency patient, the airway must be accessed initially. If the patient is obtunded or not maintaining a patent airway, the resulting hypoxia and hypercapnia will both independently contribute to increased ICP. Placement of a secure airway with an endotracheal tube must be done first, with care not to lower blood pressure and worsen CPP. In any patient with a GCS of 8 or less, intubation is indicated. If time permits, a brief neurological examination should be performed prior to administration of sedative and paralytic agents. For patients with trauma, the cervical spine must be protected from further injury through maintenance of in-line stabilization. Standard techniques of rapid sequence intubation are preferred, with pretreatment with intravenous lidocaine (1.5–2 mg/kg IV) and fentanyl (3 μg/kg IV) prior to laryngoscopy. Lidocaine and fentanyl offer the theoretical advantage of blunting laryngeal stimulation (which can lead to further increases in ICP) caused by intubation. Inductions agents must be selected and dosed appropriately to minimize the risk of transient medication-induced hypotension. Typical induction agents include thiopental (3–5 mg/kg IV) or etomidate (0.3 mg/kg IV). Because thiopental may depress cardiac output, thiopental should be avoided in patients who are hypotensive or a smaller dose used (0.5–1 mg/kg). Ketamine should be avoided as it increases ICP.

Short-acting paralytics should also be used, most commonly succinylcholine (1–2 mg/kg IV) or rocuronium (0.6–1 mg/kg IV). Because succinylcholine may lead to brief increases in ICP, some physicians prefer to pretreat with a small, defasciculating dose of vecuronium (0.01 mg/kg IV) several minutes prior to administration of succinylcholine. For patients suspected of having elevated ICP, the endotracheal tube should be secured to the face only using adhesive tape. Standard trach ties should be avoided, because a circular neck dressing may impede venous outflow from the head, promoting vascular congestion, and further elevating ICP.

Goals of mechanical ventilation should include prevention of hypoxemia and normalization of hypercapnea. As a result, during the initial resuscitation, 100 percent FiO2 should be administered. Prophylactic hyperventilation should be avoided, as it may promote intracerebral vasoconstriction and exacerbate neuronal ischemia. The goal PaCO2 should be 35–40 mmHg. Adequate sedation is critical, because asynchronous respiratory efforts while on the ventilator may cause gagging and coughing, with resulting spikes in ICP. Although sedation is initially titrated, it may be necessary to provide temporary paralysis, although paralysis eliminates the ability to follow any changes in the neurological examination. Positive end-expiratory pressure (PEEP) should be used judiciously because high PEEP may increase intrathoracic pressure, impeding venous return from the head and resulting in increased ICP.

Attention must also be directed to the patient's hemodynamic status. Hypotension should be strictly avoided in patients suspected of having increased ICP, because hypotension reduces cerebral perfusion pressure (CPP). Administration of intravenous fluids (IVF) should be the initial maneuver to maintain MAP > 90 mmHg. In cases where IVF alone is insufficient, vasopressor agents, such as dopamine or norepinephrine, may be required. Phenylephrine may also be used, although it may diminish cardiac output and result in reduced cerebral blood flow. Similarly, if blood pressure is markedly elevated, this may contribute to a pathologic state of cerebral edema and mass effect worsening and should be controlled conservatively.

General Precautions for Increased ICP

Once the ABCs have been addressed and stabilized, simple prophylactic measures should be instituted to optimize venous outflow from the head and avoid further intracranial venous congestion. These measures include keeping the head midline, avoiding any *circumferential* neck dressings, and avoiding insertion of internal jugular (IJ) central venous catheters into the dominant IJ. The Trendelenburg position should not be used (for placement of

219

central lines, etc.) as it promotes intracranial venous congestion and may increase ICP. If dangerously elevated ICP is suspected and central access is needed, it may be best to place a temporary femoral venous catheter until an ICP monitor is placed or the condition is otherwise treated, thereby initially avoiding placing a patient in the Trendelenburg position. Furthermore, using ultrasound guidance may decrease the need for Trendelenberg positioning. Patients suspected of having elevated ICP, and who are not hypotensive (MAP > 90 mmHg), should have the head of the bed raised to 30°. Initial medical interventions to help treat elevations in ICP include avoidance of exacerbating factors, such as fever, seizures, venous outflow obstruction, hyperglycemia, hypoxemia, hypercarbia or persistent vomiting.

Once the ABCs have been stabilized, an emergent noncontrast head CT should be obtained on any patient suspected of having elevated ICP. Neurosurgical and neurology consultation should be requested urgently. More specific interventions should then be initiated, such as administration of osmotic agents, induction of pharmacologic coma, and possibly therapeutic hypothermia. Neurosurgical interventions, such as placement of ICP monitors or decompressive craniotomy, may also be required.

Mannitol

Mannitol is an osmotically active agent that has long been used in the management of elevated ICP. The mechanism of its action involves multifactorial means to lower ICP, and its effectiveness in reducing ICP is well described. Decreases in ICP by approximately 20 to 35 percent within 10 to 20 minutes of intravenous administration are reported. The ICP reduction effect of mannitol typically lasts two hours. Mannitol infusion can result in an osmotic diuresis leading to hypovolemia, an undesirable effect and a poor method of attempting to treat elevated ICP. In fact, the hypovolemia that can sometimes be a consequence of mannitol therapy must be avoided because this may worsen outcomes, especially in the setting of head trauma. It is advisable, therefore, to maintain euvolemia and replace any vigorous urine output from a mannitol induced dieresis.

Mannitol should be given intravenously in a bolus dose via a peripheral or central intravenous line at a dose of 0.25 to 1.0 gram per kilogram (g/kg). Serum osmolality should be monitored, and a value of 320 mOsm/L is generally accepted as treatment endpoint. Bolus doses of mannitol are favored over continuous infusions.

Hypertonic Saline (HTS)

HTS provides another option for hyperosmolar therapy. Options include either 2%, 3%, 7.5%, or 23.4% HTS. Recent evidence supports the use of bolus doses of 30 to 60 ml of 23.4% HTS via a central line to emergently reverse a herniation event. HTS may also have a longer duration of action on ICP than mannitol. It should be emphasised that 23.4% HTS *must be administered via a central venous line* over *10–15 minutes* to prevent hypotension and phlebitis.

Infusions of lower concentrations of HTS can be used to maintain an osmotic gradient with serum sodium levels 145 to 155 mEq/L. Infusions of 2% HTS can be easily given via a peripheral line, but 3% HTS requires central access, something that should be considered if a patient has the clinical potential for cerebral herniation. Prolonged infusions of HTS will require a 50%:50% mix of sodium chloride and sodium acetate so as to prevent hyperchloremic metabolic acidosis. The infusion rate is set based on a particular patient's osmotic and intravascular needs, with typical maintenance rates of 75 ml/hr being used. If needed, these solutions can be administered in 250 milliliter boluses to treat episodes of intracranial hypertension or systemic hypotension. Frequent monitoring of serum sodium should be performed, with clear goals of treatment specified. Rapid drops in serum sodium are to be avoided so as not to precipitate cerebral edema, and rapid increases in serum sodium are likewise to be avoided in any patient with severe chronic hyponatremia in order to avoid central pontine myelinolysis.

Pharmacologic Coma to Reduce ICP

If ICP remains poorly controlled after osmotic therapy has been initiated, then induced pharmacologic coma can be considered for patients with the possibility of neurologic viability. It is thought that the effect of pharmacologic coma on ICP is through reduction of cerebral metabolism ($CMRO_2$) with reductions in cerebral blood flow (CBF) and reduced tissue oxygen demand. Pentobarbital is the most commonly used agent for pharmacological coma. This drug can be administered intravenously at a loading dose of 5 mg/kg, followed by an infusion of 1–3 mg/kg/hr. The drug is titrated to the therapeutic goals of burst suppression on continuous electroencephalography (EEG) monitoring or a reduction in ICP. If burst suppression is not obtained with this dose, then a smaller loading dose and increased rate can be given until a satisfactory EEG tracing is seen or ICP is controlled. Thiopental, a shorter acting barbiturates may be used, whose half-life of five hours is suited for short-term therapy of elevations in ICP and as a test dose to see if a patient with increased ICP may be susceptible to barbiturates. Doses of 200–500 mg of this drug can be given via bolus intravenous push while monitoring for hypotension. Complications of barbiturate use include:

- Loss of neurologic exam (except pupillary response)
- Myocardial depression and systemic hypotension
- Ileus and feeding intolerance

- Decreased mucociliary clearance (ventilator associated pneumonia)
- Occult sepsis

If pharmacologic coma is successful in attenuating ICP, then several days of such therapy is warranted, perhaps bridging the patient through a period of his maximal cerebral edema. Withdrawal of the barbiturate infusion can then be done while monitoring for subsequent rebound rises in ICP.

Propofol provides another option for pharmacological coma, and is given at an intravenous loading dose of 2 mg/kg, followed by a titrated infusion of up to 100 mcg/kg/min. The use of propofol for the treatment of refractory elevations of ICP is quite controversial. Long-term and high-dose propofol infusions have been associated with the development of a newly described metabolic disorder termed propofol infusion syndrome (PRIS). Renal failure, rhabdomyolysis, hyperkalemia, myocardial failure, metabolic acidosis, lipemia, hepatomegaly, and, in most cases, death complete this syndrome. The mechanism is not completely described, but, in light of published accounts of PRIS, caution must be used in any infusion over 5 mg/kg/hr or treatment lasting longer than 48 hours. As with the barbituates, continuous EEG monitoring is helpful to define an endpoint of a burst suppression pattern and/or ICP control.

Box 10.5 Important Point: Propofol Infusion Syndrome (PRIS)

- Prolonged infusions of propofol may be associated with a severe metabolic acidosis.
- Renal and cardiac failure, hyperkalemia, and death may follow.
- Avoid large dose or prolonged infusions of propofol, if possible.
- Strongly consider monitoring patients receiving propofol infusions with serial serum lactic acid levels, CK, LFTs, triglycerides, and troponins.

Seizure Prophylaxis

Seizure prophylaxis, with agents such as levetiracetam (500 mg PO/IV bid) or phenytoin (10–15 mg/kg IV load), is often considered early because seizure activity is associated with increased metabolic activity of the brain. Because patients with elevated ICP have a limited ability to meet increased metabolic demand, seizure activity can result in neuronal ischemia and cell death. This is usually the case in patients with large cortical lesions. However, routine use of seizure prophylaxis is debatable, as there is evidence to suggest that prophylactic use of antiepileptics could have harmful cognitive effects. If there is concern that an occult nonconvulsive seizure may be complicating the neurologic exam, then consideration should be made for administration of an anticonvulsant agent such as those just listed. This can be given for the short term and electroencephalography (EEG) studies obtained in the intensive care unit. The duration of such therapy in the setting of severe closed-head injury is much debated, but should generally be given for seven days. The use of anticonvulsants in penetrating brain injury is sustained for a longer period of time.

Induced Hypothermia

Induced hypothermia for control of elevated ICP remains quite controversial. Induced mild hypothermia (33 to 35°C) may improve outcomes as far out as two years in the setting of ICP elevations associated with head trauma, but it is unclear if this will generalize to all patients with elevated ICP, and the long-term outcome benefit remains debated. If utilized in refractory increased ICP, modalities of induction of hypothermia include skin-applied gel cooling systems and intravenous methods, as well as traditional air-circulating cooling blankets, iced gastric lavage, and surface ice packing. If this is undertaken, vigilance for complications of hypothermia including coagulopathy and occult sepsis must remain high. For the purposes of this review, it is prudent to maintain emphasis on normothermia and avoidance of fever during the initial management of increased ICP. Induced hypothermia may be considered in refractory cases and only after other means of controlling ICP have been exhausted. Further research on this area is needed and is underway.

Lumbar Puncture and Extraventricular Drainage

Lumbar Puncture (LP)

Lumbar puncture provides the safest and most successful access to sample the CSF in most patients. Removal of CSF from the lumbar cistern is contraindicated in the setting of coagulopathy, impending cerebral herniation, signs of elevated ICP on brain imaging or fundoscopy, a focal neurologic examination, or a known space occupying lesion with evidence of midline shift or subfalcine herniation. Judgment must be exercised if the positioning or time required for the lumbar puncture may aggravate an ongoing or competing respiratory or hemodynamic issue.

Ideally, the LP should be performed in the proper positioning for assessment of the opening pressure, which is an accurate assessment (in cm/H_2O) of intracranial pressure. In order to obtain an accurate measurement, the patient must be in the lateral recumbent position and have the abdomen relaxed and legs extended when the manometer reading is taking place. For some patients, particularly those who are obese, it may be difficult or impossible to perform an LP while the patient is placed in the lateral position. In these cases, the spinal needle can be introduced while the patient is in the seated position; once the lumbar cistern is entered, the patient can be carefully rotated into the lateral position for measurement of opening pressure. Some authorities recommend removing 2 cc of CSF for testing and then moving the patient flat, to ensure that some fluid is obtained. Elevations in pressure are represented by readings of over 18 –20 cm/H_2O. CSF should always be sent for analysis, including routine chemistries, cell count with differential, Gram stain, and culture.

Extraventricular Drain (EVD)

The management of elevated ICP is of paramount importance in the care of many patients with neurologic emergencies. If elevations in ICP progress unchecked, this can culminate in cerebral herniation. All patients with suspected elevation of ICP should be considered candidates for placement of an ICP monitor. Options include an intraventricular catheter (IVC) (synonymous with the extraventricular drain /EVD), intraparenchymal fiberoptic or solid state monitor, subdural bolt, and epidural fiber optic catheter. The most invasive and most accurate is the EVD, which is placed via a Burr hole into the third ventricle. The EVD also provides a treatment option for ICP management with removal of supratentorial CSF. If there is anticipation of requiring supratentorial CSF removal or hydrocephalus is seen radiographically, an EVD is the best option for monitoring ICP.

Indications for placing an ICP monitor include one of the following:

• A patient with a GCS score < eight (after resuscitation)
• An acute abnormality on CT

Or a patient with two of the following:

• SBP < 90 mmHg
• Motor posturing on exam
• ≥ 40 years of age

If the preceding conditions are met, then an ICP monitor should be placed or strongly considered. These indications refer specifically to patients in the setting of trauma, but are utilized in the setting of severe neurologic injury or when the neurologic exam is poor and elevations in ICP are suspected or likely.

Decompressive Craniectomy

Decompressive craniectomy (DC) is an aggressive, although effective treatment for intractable elevations in ICP. DC has been utilized in the setting of head trauma, intracerebral hemorrhage, hemispheric ischemic stroke, among other indications. The reported experience to date is conflicting, although currently there are two randomized controlled trials ongoing currently for the study of DC in head trauma. Early decompressive craniectomy may obviate the need to use more conventional methods to control ICP, such as pharmacological coma, and may exist as a therapeutic option in the setting of intractable elevations in ICP in an otherwise salvageable patient. New data exists to support hemicraniectomy in the setting of ICP elevations from hemispheric stroke, and consultation with a neurosurgeon with this in mind may be warranted in this and other such cases.

Key Points:

- Hydrocephalus may represent a neurologic emergency depending on the tempo of its development; acute hydrocephalus requires immediate intervention to prevent neurologic injury.

- IIH should not be considered a benign illness, and neurologic and ophthalmologic evaluation should be sought when IIH is suspected.

- Intracranial hypotension from spontaneous CSF leaks is a cause of postural headache and SDH.

- In patients with CSF shunts, evaluate patency or efficiency of drainage (over or under) in all cases presenting with new headache, fever, focal neurologic deficits, or altered mental status.

- Maintain a high index of suspicion for elevated ICP in patients with poor neurologic examinations in the setting of an acute intracranial mass lesion.

- Cerebral herniation syndrome may occur in the absence of elevated ICP.

- Be familiar with surgical and medical means to treat increased ICP and reverse a potential herniation syndrome.

- Patients with concern or evidence of increased ICP or processes that may result in elevated ICP are best monitored in the neurosciences critical-care unit or ICU, until a period of stability has been achieved.

Suggested Reading

Blumenfeld H. *Neuroanatomy through Clinical Cases.* Sunderland, MA: Sinauer Associates, Inc.; 2002:137–151.

Brazis PW, Masdeu JC, Biller J. *Localization in Clinical Neurology.* Philadelphia: Lippincott Williams and Wilkins; 2007:521–555.

Bullock MR, Chesnut R, Ghajar J, et al. Surgical management of traumatic parenchymal lesions. *Neurosurgery.* 2006;58(3 Suppl):S25–S46.

Campbell WW. *Dejong's the Neurologic Examination*. Philadelphia: Lippincott Williams and Wilkins; 2005:597–601.

Cutler RW, Page L, Galichich J, et al. Formation and absorption of cerebrospinal fluid in man. *Brain*. 1968;91(4):707–720.

Greenberg MS. *Handbook of Neurosurgery*. New York: Thieme; 2006:171–204.

Hofmeijer J, Kappelle LJ, Algra A, et al. Surgical decompression for space-occupying cerebral infarction (the Hemicraniectomy After Middle Cerebral Artery infarction with Life-threatening Edema Trial [HAMLET]): a multicentre, open, randomised trial. *Lancet Neurol*. 2009;8(4):326–333. Epub 2009; Mar 5.

Koenig MA, Bryan M, Lewin JL 3rd, Mirski MA, Geocadin RG, Stevens RD. Reversal of transtentorial herniation with hypertonic saline. *Neurology*. 2008 Mar 25;70(13):1023–1029.

Ling GS, Marshall SA. Management of traumatic brain injury in the intensive care unit. *Neurol Clin*. 2008;26(2):409–426.

Oddo M, Levine JM, Frangos S, et al. Effect of mannitol and hypertonic saline on cerebral Oxygenation in patients with severe traumatic brain injury and refractory intracranial hypertension. *J Neurol Neurosurg Psychiatry*. 2009;80:916–920.

Povlishock JT, Bratton SL, Randall M, et al. Guidelines for the management of severe traumatic brain injury. *J Neurotrauma*. 2007;24(Suppl 1):S1–S95.

Prabhakar H, Umesh G, Chouhan RS, Bithal PK. Reverse brain herniation during posterior fossa surgery. *J Neurosurg Anesthesiol*. 2003;15(3):267–269.

Qiu WS, Liu WG, Shen H, et al. Therapeutic effect of mild hypothermia on severe traumatic head injury. *Chin J Traumatol*. 2005;8(1):27–32.

Qiu WS, Liu WG, Shen H, et al. Therapeutic effect of mild hypothermia on severe traumatic head injury. *Chin J Traumatol*. 2005;8:27-32.Randhawa S, Van Stavern GP. Idiopathic intracranial hypertension (pseudotumor cerebri). *Curr Opin Ophthalmol*. 2008;19(6):445–453.

Raslan A, Bhardwaj A. Medical management of cerebral edema. *Neurosurg Focus*. 2007;22(5):E12.

Rasomoff H. Methods of simultaneous quantitative estimation of intracranial contents. *J Appl Physiol*. 1953;16:395–396.

Ratanalert SN, Phuenpathom N, Saeheng S, et al. ICP threshold in CPP management of severe head injury patients. *Surg Neurol*. 2004;61:429–435.

Schievink W. Spontaneous spinal CSF leaks and intracranial hypotension. *JAMA*. 2006;295:2286–2296.

Smith H, Sinson G, Varelas P. Vasopressors and propofol infusion syndrome in severe head trauma. *Neurocrit Care*. 2009;10(2):166–172.Vilela MD. Delayed paradoxical herniation after a decompressive craniectomy: case report. *Surg Neurol*. 2008;69:293–296.

Ware ML, Nemani VM, Meeker M, Lee C, Morabito DJ, Manley GT. Effects of 23.4% sodium chloride solution in reducing intracranial pressure in patients with traumatic brain injury: a preliminary study. *Neurosurgery*. 2005;57:727–736.

Yang XF, Wen L, Shen L, et al. Surgical complications secondary to decompressive craniectomy in patients with a head injury: a series of 108 consecutive cases. *Acta Neurochir (Wien)*. 2008;150(12):1241–1247.

Index

Note: Page references followed by "*f*" and "*t*" denote figures and table, respectively.

227